The Phoenix Rises

Lockdown Chronicles

The Phoenix Rises

Lockdown Chronicles

Editor
Amit Dasgupta

wisdom tree

ISBN: 978-81-8328-564-3

Published by
Wisdom Tree
4779/23, Ansari Road
Darya Ganj, New Delhi-110 002
Ph.: 011-23247966/68
wisdomtreebooks@gmail.com

Printed in India

Dedicated to survival
and the unbreakable human spirit

'There's a crack in everything
And that's how the light gets in'

—LEONARD COHEN

The *Phoenix* is a mythical bird, symbolising immortality,
as it rises from the ashes of its predecessor.

Contents

Lockdown Litfest: Coronavirus Curfew Could Give Rise to a Whole New Literary Genre

Jug Suraiya

The politically repressive Soviet regime gave rise to an underground literature of resistance against dictatorial authority. Dissidents would copy or compose essays, stories, poems against state censorship.

These writings were given the collective name *samizdat*, which in Russian means 'self-published'. As typewriters and other printing devices had to be officially registered, these manuscripts were all handwritten and passed on from reader to reader.

As one exponent of the genre noted, 'I write by myself. I edit by myself. I publish by myself. I distribute by myself. And I shall go to prison by myself.'

The *samizdat* was a secret weapon in a war of liberation. Today, in the midst of the Coronavirus pandemic, not just one country but the whole world is engaged in a far more deadly war of freedom—freedom from the invisible, all-pervasive death-dealing spectre of COVID-19.

Like all wars, this war too has its heroes—the doctors

and health workers—who have put themselves in the front line of greatest danger. The war has its martyrs—the hundreds of thousands who have succumbed to the deadly disease, and it has its collateral damage in the migrant labourers and others who have lost their livelihoods and are facing brute poverty.

It is a unique war, a war without frontiers. For the first time, humanity is facing a fight to the finish, which does not divide it into opposing factions but unifies it against a common foe.

And while across the globe we desperately search for a protective shield against this implacable enemy, the universal lockdown has inspired an avatar of the Soviet-era *samizdat*, as people across the planet in curfew-bound isolation make communion with each other—and with themselves—by written and spoken reflections on the pandemic and what it means to them, and what it might mean for the world of tomorrow.

A friend, Amit Dasgupta, is compiling an e-book of personalised accounts of people's experiences and emotions at this time of unprecedented crisis. A chiaroscuro of light and dark, of hope and fear, of loss and longing, such projects can stand as enduring testaments to the resilience of the human spirit, uniting us as we have never been before.

That is the tragic triumph of humanity over the virus.

This article was originally printed in *The Times of India*.

'Now I am become Death,
the destroyer of worlds'

—BHAGVAD GITA

Introduction

'There's a loneliness in this world so great that you can see it in the slow movement of the hands of a clock.'

— CHARLES BUKOWSKI

The pandemic has dramatically disrupted life the world over. It is said that nothing, as we knew it, would ever be the same. Our vocabulary has already incorporated words like 'contagion', 'social distancing', 'herd immunity', 'lockdown' and many others as common parlance. We work from home and carry out our professional meetings virtually. Travelling, shopping, a visit to the grocery store or vegetable market, an after-office drink with friends, a visit to the cinema or a restaurant would now need to be planned and coordinated well in advance. Whims and on-the-spur-of-the-moment decisions would be a thing of the past. A life we once knew and had taken for granted is over. This is the 'new normal' that would control and dominate our social, personal and professional lives. Worse, it is not temporary.

As the country went into lockdown mode from end of March, it would be fair to say that there was widespread confusion and uncertainty with each extension of the lockdown. This is understandable. For a country of 1.3 billion people, with high population density, it was eerie to see empty streets, shut shops, police patrols and border control, on the rare occasion one left home for medicines or groceries. The entire neighbourhood looked like a ghost town. No stray dogs either. An occasional crow, perhaps. We find it difficult to fathom because we are a socially gregarious people used to hustle-bustle and crowds. All of a sudden, we found ourselves enveloped by an impenetrable silence and emptiness. It was as if Death had wandered in and decided to stay.

Some said 2020 was a bad year. A really bad year and as close to *Kaliyug* as possible. It was predicted, we were informed, in ancient scriptures thousands of years ago and by Nostradamus himself about its coming. Many turned to prayer and chanting. Several others to WhatsApp. Experts mushroomed. The media carried opinion pieces. Television debates raged. The virus was dissected and analysed, and advisories issued. Each differed widely from the other. No one genuinely seemed to have a clue as to what was actually going on. The Internet was filled with horrific images of a convoy of coffins in Iran silently making its way through empty streets, or the dead and dying in China and Indonesia, or the number of fatalities in the US, or the quarantine of a prime minister, and much more. This was the tapestry of our daily information updates. We watched our neighbours with suspicion. If we needed to leave the safety of our home, we wore masks and stood well apart from other people. It left us distressed and confused, because this, we told ourselves, is not us. Panic set in. And fear, which we all knew was contagious. Things would only get worse.

When the lockdown was first imposed, it was seen as a novelty. A friend referred to it as a picnic at home with the family on a weekday. With no cars or buses on the streets, pollution levels dramatically dropped. As the days wore on, forest animals wandered on to the city streets and the empty marketplaces. It was extraordinary and fascinating. I wrote a short article describing this and was surprised at the effusive reaction of many, who shared their personal experiences.

In the early weeks, the experience was entirely driven by a sense of novelty. Many tried their hand at things they had never tried before, such as, cooking or painting. WhatsApp was flooded with photographs of last night's dinner and the ooohs and aaahs from friends was pleasurable. But, as the lockdown period extended, many complained of boredom, even loneliness. The positives vanished and a shroud of gloom, a sense of uncertainty and negativity characterised our daily lives.

This is certainly an extraordinary time. The first in our lifetime and in any case, the biggest lockdown in global history. I discussed with Shobit Arya, the publisher, and the idea of capturing the varied reactions in a compilation took shape. The speed with which the persons we reached out to responded was an endorsement that there was indeed a story that needed to be captured and shared.

This volume is by no means complete nor, indeed, could it have hoped to be. Many stories are conspicuous by their absence. For instance, stories of persons who contracted the virus and recovered. Or of those who did not. The suffering of their families and especially, the lonely last journey to the funeral pyre. Or stories of extraordinary courage and sacrifice from innumerable doctors, nurses and frontline health workers, of journalists, who covered the story fearlessly on a daily basis, of security and administration officials, who worked long and thankless hours for days on end. Of separated families with no hope of reuniting during the lockdown, of the elderly, who had to manage on their own. Of children, who could not understand what was happening and why they could no longer go out to play with their friends or had to study at home. Of the several thousand small businesses that were forced to close shop. Or of the many who lost jobs. Or stories of community workers, NGOs and common people, who reached out to assist the needy, the elderly, the infirm and the impoverished. Their stories have not been told in this volume.

Nor indeed, is the plight of the migrants, the poor and the marginalised adequately captured in the volume. When hundreds of thousands of them spilled over onto our streets and then, began the long march home, many barefoot, there was an overwhelming shock and surprise. Where did they come from? It appeared as if no one, not even the government and local administration, was aware of their existence! And yet, we had seen and interacted with them on a daily basis. As security guards in the gated communities and housing societies we lived in, as domestic help, as vegetable vendors and waiters and cooks in restaurants, as mechanics in the auto and bicycle repair shops, as ticket collectors in buses and the metro station, as auto and taxi drivers. They were all around us and yet, we failed to take note of their existence.

They came from places as distant as Bihar and Bengal, Odisha, Assam and Karnataka. All they wanted was to go back home. Horrific images circulated in the national and social media of men and women, carrying infants, of bleeding feet that were cracked and burnt by the melting tar in the blazing summer heat. Images of people desperately trying to scramble on to packed buses and lorries with an infant, precariously, cradled in one hand. Many died. What happened will be a national shame. As a government and as a people, we disowned and abandoned, nay, betrayed our own for, as Borges so aptly put it,

'We rob him of everything,
we leave him not so much as a colour or syllable:
here, the courtyard which his eyes no longer see,
there, the sidewalk where his hope lay in wait.'

For this and several other reasons, the volume is inadequate and incomplete. It fails to fully capture the extraordinary and turbulent time we are all passing through. Perhaps a year or so later, when things, hopefully, might have settled down, another volume could, would and certainly, should be put together that can more comprehensively document the stories, the reflections, the tragedy and finally, the aftermath of a time that was. It is possible that an antidote would have been found by then and we would declare victory over the pandemic and the healing process would begin. It would, however, be a tragedy if, by then, we fail to learn how more lives could have been saved and how we might have done things better.

But, till then, I do believe that this volume reflects the sentiments and emotions of many fellow travellers and I am glad that it has been possible to put it together.

II

There are many I need to thank. Shobit is at the top of the list. For a publisher to take a gamble, especially at a time like this, is either a reflection of extreme naivety or visionary imagination. Shobit has published some of my earlier books and I have full faith that he believes this volume to be timely.

To Jug Suraiya, a friend of many years, whose writing so many of us have loved and admired, I owe a deep sense of gratitude. Not only has Jug shared his thoughts and reflections in the volume but he went the extra mile and wrote about the book in his popular column in *The Times of India*. That led to a number of his friends reaching out with their contributory articles and this truly became a book of reflections from friends and friends of friends. For that I am deeply grateful. A bonus came along in the form of a contributory article from Jug's lovely wife, Bunny. I could not have asked for more and was confident that the book was well on its way.

Almost everyone I reached out to, agreed to write

and they did. They came from different professions. Journalists, doctors, school teachers, authors, first-time writers. I loved reading their thoughts and reflections and believe that each contributory piece added value and brought in new insights.

My gratitude to each and every one of the contributors: Amrita Narayanan, Anita Anand, Anjum Katyal, Antara Dev Sen, Anuradha Kumar, Avijit Dutt, Beetashok Chatterjee, Bunny Suraiya, Debi Mukhopadhyay, Deepak Hiranandani, Deepak Sanan, Dilip Bobb, J. Alfred Prufrock, Jael Silliman, Jayshree Misra Tripathi, Jug Suraiya, Lakshmi Subramanian, Lalita Panicker, Mangala Gouri Chakraborty, Mitra Phukan, Mousumi Sengupta, Nandini Dutta, Navtej Sarna, Nikita Bathla, Papia Roy, Pooja Poddar Marwah, Randhir Khare, Reena I. Puri, Snigdha Agrawal, Sohan Hatangadi, Sumit Mullick, Sunil Gupta, Sunita Biswas, Supriya Newar, Sushmita Bose, Tsering Gellek, Tuktuk Ghosh.

III

Discussions have already commenced as to what a post-pandemic world would look like and even what it *should* look like. Economists predict that it would take quite a while for the world to come out of its comatose state. Sociologists predict social upheaval. Others predict a rise in mental health issues, including acute depression and even suicide. There are so many different points of view that it is difficult to make sense of what the future holds in store. Most of us would simply wish to get on with our lives and do what we were used to. Our life, as we knew it, gave us a sense of comfort because we knew what to expect. It was predictable. The pandemic took that away from us and that is why we were unnerved and confused. We want that feeling of comfort back. Our concern is really with what happens to us. If social upheavals and an economic slowdown affect our everyday lives in a negative way, we would feel concerned. If not, we would leave it to those who wish to pontificate in newspapers or through television debates. The concern for the poor and the deprived was never central to our personal agenda. Unless we are directly affected, we would prefer not to be involved.

What we do know now about the pandemic is that it affects people in different ways. For most, the pandemic has been an irritant and a terrible inconvenience. For the poor and the migrant workers, it has been a loss of livelihood and thus, a matter of survival. Recent developments suggest that people are increasingly willing to unite and protest against injustice. The mass rallies in the US to protest against racial abuse and brutality reflect this. The horrors of colonialism would no longer be glorified, as was seen through recent events in Europe. Governments are increasingly coming to recognise that post-pandemic governance would necessarily need to be far more inclusive and based on the principle that the poor matter.

The transition from a 'me' society to a 'we' society lies at the heart of democratic governance, though it has long been elusive. It needs to be driven by people rather than governments. Perhaps, it is an idea whose time has come.

A gentler, kinder society that deviates from the old ways of doing things to new ways of seeing things. When that happens and I believe it will, the Phoenix will rise from the ashes.

Noida
June 2020

AMIT DASGUPTA

Present Tense

Jug Suraiya

Like many, if not most people, I didn't live my life so much as I planned on living it. I was always busy making plans about what I was going to do.

Short-term plans, like which place to go eat out on the coming weekend. Medium-term plans, like where to go for the summer holiday. Long-term plans, like what new investment to make when an old investment matured next year.

I was like a traveller whose eyes are fixed on the distant horizon ahead, and who is oblivious of his immediate surroundings, the ground underfoot, the gritty rasp of concrete, or the smooth spring of grass, the roar of city traffic around or the singing silence of open spaces, the urban jostle of steel and glass or the murmurous green of wind-sighing trees.

If I noticed all this, it was through peripheral vision, trapped as I was in the confines of a calendar, which dictated to me the things I had to do, or wanted to do, in the time yet to come.

And in living in this time yet to come, without knowing or realising it, I was losing out on the present.

When we anticipate a happiness or a hardship to come, today's joys and sorrows fleet by us, as insubstantial as a dream being dreamt by another. Then, like a camera coming into sudden focus so that a hazy picture jumps into sharp clarity, the Coronavirus effect thrust the present on us in all its bristling immediacy.

No more envisioning things and events a week, a month, a year to come. Part of it, of course, was the lockdown, which squeezed time and space into the cramped claustrophobia of curfew. But even after the lockdown ends, the uncharted and unchartable course of the pandemic would have scattered all our carefully-made plans to the random winds of chance.

The virus has given us a gift, the gift of the present. Whether it's a welcome or unwelcome gift is up to us. But the present, tense as it may be, is all we have. Or ever had.

Homeward Bound

Jug Suraiya

Bunny and I have recently discovered the small terrace adjoining our bedroom on the first floor. It's always been there for all the past twenty-four years that we've been living in this house, of course, and every now and then we would look at it and wonder what we could do with it.

For most parts of the year, Gurugram, where we live, is either too hot or too cold for us to use the terrace as a sit-out. We could have turned it into an extra room, but we don't need more enclosed space. So, the terrace lay there like a fallow field—unproductive and useless.

Then came the Coronavirus lockdown, and because of it we discovered our long-neglected terrace. Unable to leave home because of the curfew, we began to use our terrace for our daily evening walk of forty-five minutes. Our white elephant of a terrace became a godsend.

Like us, a lot of people all over the world are making all sorts of happy discoveries in their homes. These needn't be as large as a tiny terrace—ours is 20 feet by 15 feet. Indeed, some of these chance findings could be small, like a discarded, frayed rug unearthed at random from the recesses of a cupboard and which becomes a handy yoga mat, to help keep you fit during the lockdown.

It could be a book you'd bought, but forgotten to read, a DVD you'd got but never watched. It might be a bottle of sauce, or a jar of a condiment you come across while rummaging through the kitchen cabinet and which inspires a new, tasty twist to an old recipe to help dispel Corona blues. But perhaps the best thing we have discovered about our homes, which we take so much for granted that we overlook or fail to appreciate about them, is how lucky we are to have a home to call our own, while millions of our fellow citizens live on the pavements or in makeshift shanties.

There's an old saying, *'Ghar ki murgi, daal barabar'*, which roughly translates as, 'Even something special made at home becomes ordinary.' Today that should be inverted to, *'Ghar ki daal, murgi barabar.'*

Unprecedented

Sunita Biswas

Perhaps this is what a siege felt like in the past with the enemy at the gates?

Only this time around, the enemy is invisible. And the gates are everywhere!

Or a bomb-shelter? Waiting for the all-clear to ring. Only no one knows when!

Unprecedented: our locked-down lives.

Unprecedented: people, who were a part of our daily existence, suddenly vanished, and the virtual became our only reality. A new set of instructions advise us how to live our lives: avoid people!

Unprecedented in the way we quickly adopted a whole new jargon to understand and explain the altered realities. Social distancing. Shelter in place. Contact tracing. Immuno-compromised. Herd immunity.

Unprecedented in the anxiety and uncertainty about oneself and loved ones. In the redefining of relationships and the meaning of home and the blessings of the indoors. In the awareness of the difference between real and felt needs.

Unprecedented in the way people have found all kinds of ways to inspire and reassure the world.

That this masked existence too shall pass and we shall overcome.

The First Line of Defence: In Pursuit of Health and Humanity

Nikita Bathla

If you ever ask a doctor why they chose to be one, the answer you will get will always be a version of 'I want to make a difference.' As young medical students, we learn the definitions of 'outbreak', 'epidemic' and 'pandemic', never fully absorbing what they mean. We discuss yellow fever in Africa, the plague in Europe and dengue in Asia and they always seem too far away, or too long ago. We move along our medical careers narrowing our perspectives from the population to the patient, focusing on making every person we encounter healthy. As years go by, we are fascinated with the advances in technology to aid us in our practice. We continuously upskill ourselves—a doctor can never stop learning. We become more and more specialised; there is little modern medicine cannot achieve.

Then one day we hear of a virus originating in Wuhan, China. Experts christen it 'novel', something we've never seen before. We hear titbits of information daily, on news channels and social media. Just enough to spark our interest, not enough to worry about. We know that this time it may be different, a respiratory virus on a rampage. The possibilities are endless. Infectivity and transmission are simple concepts we had learned as young medical students. We reminisce about Ebola, and how the world rallied together to contain it. Our faith in modern medicine and the global health workforce is unrelenting. We think of our world, more connected than ever. Will our connectivity spell doom?

As weeks pass, the situation seems more dire. Countries are halting flights and sealing borders as cases continue to rise. They appear as red dots on a world map, spreading like wildfire. First, the panic sets in. How will we cope? With more than 1.3 billion people, the situation in India is more vulnerable than ever. We know better than anyone what our health system can take. Countries start to take stock of their doctors and nurses, hospital beds and ventilators. We bid farewell and distance ourselves from our families, not wanting to expose our loved ones to our occupational hazards. We realise we are not prepared; we're reacting. We think, we'll make do with our limited resources, as we have done for decades. After all, we had taken an oath—people's lives are at stake. We're ready. And then, at a moment's notice, every ward is a war zone, every health worker a warrior.

While all of the country stays locked in and protected, we work. This is why we chose this profession—to serve humanity. We had hoped it wouldn't come to this, but the time is here, to save and protect precious lives. We watch our peers being evicted and assaulted; it breaks our hearts, we are just human after all. They call us warriors, soldiers and saviours. They clap for us from their balconies and terraces. We don't hear their praises, or take note of the injustices, we just rally forward.

This virus is new, something unknown. We have to be on our toes, change tactics at a moment's notice. We've never seen such an urgency in science. We know that good science takes time. Every day we're asked, 'When will there be a vaccine?' We are the experts, the go-to people in the midst of a pandemic. And yet, there's so much we don't know. We're playing football with a moving goal post. Every day we implore our families and friends, and anyone who will listen, to stay inside, to stay safe and to conform with 'the new normal'. And every day, we put ourselves in harm's way, as we always have—for the greater good.

We count the small wins—the negative results, the discharged patients. But we never lose sight that we must continue to fight, and that this battle will be long and enduring. Some days are especially hard, when we lose a patient or one of our own. We wonder about what we could have done differently. Perhaps we should have voiced ourselves louder when we saw healthcare being sidelined for more profitable ventures. Perhaps we should have demanded laws for the rights of health workers. Perhaps we have a larger role to play than that which we've been playing. We watch how health has replaced politics on primetime news debates. We watch our peers with pride, giving their expert opinions on TV. We begin to note the inadequacies in the system that have stemmed from decades of neglect.

We all begin to question: 'Why don't we have enough protective equipment?'—we have been sent to war without ammunition. 'Why don't we have enough hospital beds?' 'Why are we being advised to take a medicine without conclusive proof that it will protect us against this virus?' As we ask these questions, as practitioners, researchers and academics, it brings us closer, we find unity in adversity. We begin to collectively remember that healthcare, our tiny niche, is bigger than us and our patients. We recall the definition of health from our middle school biology class: 'Health is not the mere absence of illness, but a state of physical, mental and social well-being.' We realise how intricately intertwined health is with politics, society and with our economy. One cannot function optimally without the other. A health crisis has brought the world to a standstill, and no amount of wealth or development has been able to deter it. We are at the frontline, which implies that we are the fingertip, the first point of contact. The decisions for healthcare are made higher up, in parliaments and ivory towers. And if we want to be able to serve our people to the best of our abilities, we must be empowered by those decisions. We believe we deserve better, and for that, we must demand and strive for better.

As the country opens up, and people begin to venture out to restart their lives, we continue our fight from the wards, the laboratories and universities. Just as every other human being, this pandemic has changed us too. It has shown us the bigger picture and urged us to prioritise healthcare for ourselves and our future generations. It has highlighted that there is no wealth without health. Through this pandemic we have donned not only our personal protective equipment in the hospitals but many other hats—of experts, leaders, health advocates, researchers and myth busters. Health is a priority now more than ever, lest we forget the far-reaching effects of the COVID-19 pandemic. We continue to work, as we always have, but with an ever-strengthened faith in science and an unwavering belief in the resilience of the human race. We transform our responsibility into power so that next time, when we act, we don't react.

Close Encounters of the Corona Kind

Anjum Katyal

Of course the ancient doomsday prophecies are being evoked: Nostradamus, the Apocalypse, *Kaliyug*. How can they not be? Flood and fire, pestilence unleashed upon the populace. Reversal of all that is seen as the natural order. The end of the world as we know it. An unprecedented pandemic, sweeping swiftly from one end of the globe to the other, striking indiscriminately at the mighty and the weak, the rich and the poor, the young and the old, regardless of race, religion, nation.

Some are seeing it as a lesson from Mother Nature. With mankind locked behind four walls, the rest of the natural world rapidly recovers the robust healthiness Homo sapiens had destroyed. Environmentalists are validated. All it takes is a few weeks without the toxic fumes and chemical poisons of urban civilisation, and we are blessed with a resurgence of blue skies, clean seas, cavorting dolphins, starry nights, singing birds and breathable air. The sparrows are back. Nothing more clearly sends out the signal that man, with his greed for more and more consumption, is the single most deadly enemy of our blue ball, this home we all share, planet Earth. Look how she blossoms without our evil interventions.

And yet, Janus-like, even as we look back at age-old scriptures and a less polluted era of simpler lifestyles, we simultaneously seem to be fast-forwarding into a world straight out of a science fiction, a world my diet of popular sci-fi paperbacks and futuristic cinema has taught me to recognise. A mutant virus that terrorises the world and has no cure. Rumoured to have been cooked in a petri dish and unleashed on humanity. Increasingly isolated lifestyles, with human interaction largely through the screen—whether it is work, shopping, recreation or intimacy. Minimum human to human contact. Robots taking over more and more everyday tasks. Technology-driven mind control directing our choices of government, music, life partner. Driverless cars and trains. Enhanced virtual reality replacing direct experience, from adventure sports to tourism. Drones monitoring the streets and public gatherings, recording minutiae which can be recalled and examined as required. Continuous surveillance of individual lives, from financial and medical details, to where we go, whom we meet and what we eat. On the one hand, choices, choices, choices. On the other, control, control, control. A seeming paradox. And somewhere in there, an attempt to understand the role, in this scenario, of that imperilled and increasingly quaint concept—freedom.

What kind of a world will we emerge into, blinking and bemused, when we are released from our protective custodies? Will it be gentler, less driven, less greedy? Will we consume, waste and pollute less, savour human contact and interaction more, be allowed a better work-life balance? Will children, heartily sick of being stuck indoors with only their mobile phones and computer screens to interface with, prefer to play outdoors and with each other? Will adults put aside their devices in favour of the face-to-face conversation of which they have been starved? All of this is possible. Or, will we walk into a much harsher, more rigid environment? Will we find ourselves submitting to escalating levels of surveillance and control by governments and corporates, in the name of our overall safety and security? Will we find authoritative decisions taken and draconian measures put in place while we focused on washing our hands and sanitising surfaces? Will we feel the loss of our individual liberty? And what then will be the fate of that quaint concept—freedom?

It remains to be seen what we, as human beings, carry out with us as lessons learned from this long lockdown. There can be no simple return to life as we knew it. Because inevitably this period of isolation and quarantine will have altered us in some way. By bringing into focus what we value, what is unnecessary to our well-being and what is essential, by forcing us to adjust our habits and lifestyle to a new situation and find out what suits us about it and what we can't stomach. In other words, we begin to understand ourselves a little better when we are pared of everything but the basics. We uncover depths, fears, talents, preferences. We are bound to emerge as changed people. Even if we return to our earlier routines, we will engage with them differently. And some of us may choose to try new things rather than go back to the way things were. Also, systems, processes and the outer world itself will have changed. There is bound to be a new normal to get used to, from something simple like wearing a mask in public to the ways in which we travel, eat out, shop.

When the lockdown began, I thought of it as an interruption, unwelcome but necessary, and reluctantly wrote it off as a time of waiting for life to resume. Soon I realised that this *was* life, and that if I didn't want days, hours and months of my remaining time on Earth to vanish into nothingness, I should start living this unexpected life as fully as possible. Despite the anxiety, the low and dull phases, the inability to focus, the weariness—which, face it, was part of my earlier life as well—I had to find meaning and value in it.

Years from now history books will mark this moment—the year 2020—as a decisive watershed in the human story. By virtue of being a truly universal experience, affecting everyone from remote Tasmania to busy New York, from celebrities in their mansions to the homeless on the streets. Months when the whole world shut down. Children will ask of their parents and grandparents—where were you when Corona hit? What was it like? What did you do?

And we have to think of how to make sense of this experience, how to process it, so that we come out of it not seeing ourselves as impoverished, diminished somehow—but differently abled, to borrow a term from another context.

Unlock Diaries

Lakshmi Subramanian

What does it feel, coming out of a lockdown? It is hard to make sense of the question for more than one reason. For one, this lockdown is different from what I have always understood the term to mean—a security measure intended to regain some control over a rapidly deteriorating situation. It was clear from the start that at no stage did anyone—state, citizen, media—have any idea about how bad the situation actually was and whether the locking down of quotidian life, as we knew it, would improve it. It also brought home to me very dramatically that at a simple level, we were locking out basic human contact in order to stay 'safe'. The latter was, in fact, a grotesque precondition—no matter how many messages exhorted us to stay apart but stay connected, there was a wave of fear and suspicion about human contact. All of a sudden, friends and strangers alike with whom I have rubbed shoulders at shop counters to get my milk, eggs and bread were to be kept at arm's length! What made the situation hard was the sense of alienation such self-conscious discipline produced. And this in a village where even in pre-COVID times, I usually met a couple of people and lots of stray dogs and cows on a five-kilometre morning walk, barring Sundays when churchgoers came out in their best attire.

But as the lockdown extended to versions 2 and then 3, the virus assumed menacing proportions for me, personally. I lost my closest friend who went without notice and without intimation. It brought home to me the fleetingness of life and the extraordinary times I am living in. This was not about looking at history being made out there, it was being part of the mess, of the sadness and the confusion and it made me even more impatient for the lockdown to lift, and for the time when I could maybe even contemplate travel. But with every passing day, I grew more unsure of whether I could actually emerge from the lockdown that had paralysed me from within.

For as I carried out my chores, telling myself that things were changing, I still felt mentally locked out. I was painfully aware of a sense of disbelief and diffidence about going back to the pre-COVID times I knew. Would I be able to go back to an easy handshake with people I barely knew; spend time talking and socialising with acquaintances without wondering whether they were asymptomatic or not; board a crowded bus without a second thought?

Yet, it is simple everyday sociality that I crave. I have never liked crowds but suddenly that seems irrelevant, for what I want, above all, is to renew my basic connection with people and engage in ordinary sociality without paranoia and inhibition. I want community—of strangers and colleagues. I want to be able to go back to campus and teach in a classroom, feasting my eyes on students, listening to them giggle, watching them yawn and occasionally argue with me. I have missed their presence in my life. It is true that virtually they have been around and have helped me transit to online teaching, which was certainly a learning experience, even if Zoom fatigue occasionally overwhelmed me.

If the classroom beckons, the archive commands. As a historian, the archive is my field and I yearn to return to it. Having scoured them all my life, I have felt strangely lost without the comfort of working amidst dusty files, or agonising over an elusive source and of hunting it down like a patient sleuth. The archive fever rages within me as I dream about a document that assumes larger than life dimensions for a facile argument that I am about to make. It is to the archive, not the healthiest of places to be, that I wish to return. As Carolyn Steedman put it so eloquently, 'Dust knows no end which cannot be dispersed, as the harbourer of the anthrax infection which also knows no end and cannot be dispersed.' I wish to say the same of the virus that stalks us today, that has robbed many of us of our dearly loved ones and for whom life is never going to be the same again. I hope I can emerge from the lockdown within me to experience life and everyday living celebrating my six senses, when I don't need to dither about buying a ticket to visit a friend, to share a hug and wipe a tear, or indeed to hide my allergic cough without obsessively checking my temperature.

Lockdown Experiences

Sunil Gupta

'If you want to be happy, do not dwell in the past, do not worry about the future, focus on living fully in the present.'

—ROY T. BENNETT, *The Light in the Heart*

I tried, people, I tried.

But unaccountably the present seems to bunch up into a smorgasbord of the past...memories, experiences, people, events, regrets, triumphs, happy times and sad times and sometimes no times at all.

Nostalgia sums it up: that's the dish on the daily menu.

And it's exemplified by my books.

Over the past few weeks, I've reordered my library (such as it is), and rediscovered a million (OK, OK about a hundred) old gems, lying dusty and forgotten, at the back of shelves, cupboards and drawers.

And in every genre: humour, thrillers, essays and anthologies, whodunits, autobiographies, bios, classics. Here is a sprinkling of the open sandwiches, all of vintage quality, from the 1950s and 60s:

George Mikes: You'd never guess he was a Hungarian self-exiled in England. His *'How to…'* (*Be Poor, Be a Brit, Be Decadent* etc.) are slim volumes packed with understated, penetrating, dry wit. It's as if he was speaking sotto voce directly to you. And that leads me to…

C. Northcote Parkinson: *Parkinson's Law,* written again with deadpan wit, should be required reading till doomsday. '*Work expands so as to fill the time available for its completion'* was as relevant seventy-five years ago as it is today and will be tomorrow. His incisive observation was based on two principles: (1) 'An official wants to multiply subordinates, not rivals,' and (2) 'Officials make work for each other.' It was written in 1958. It will be true in 2058.

Jerome K. Jerome: *Three Men in a Boat* goes even further back, to 1889. Add to it *Three Men on the Bummel* and you have a humorous duology that's timeless.

As an aside, what's with all these Brit authors? They seemed to have cornered the market for humour, for if you add PG Wodehouse, *Punch* Magazine, Stephen Fry, the earlier books of Gerald D, Christopher Matthew, even Sue Townsend, there's no one who can hold a candle to them. The secret, I think, is in their ability to find humour in anything, and to be able to cast the first joke at themselves. If only…

But the real sleeper is…

Lawrence Durrell: The Larry of Gerald Durrell's seminal, *My Family and Other Animals* was, as you would know of course, a famous author. Usually heavy stuff like *The Alexandria Quartet*. But how many know that his sense of humour was as trenchant and droll as say, a Jerome K. Jerome? His three slim volumes on the adventures of the British diplomatic corps, *Suave Qui Peut, Esprit de Corps, Stiff Upper Lip* (fictionalised, of course, but he was in the Corps himself so there's always a *soupçon* of reality), are required reading for anyone who has a penchant for real humour.

Then came the whodunits beyond *par excellence*: **Agatha Christie,** which led me to a rerun of David Suchet's incomparable portrayal of Hercule Poirot. All the others come nowhere close... Finney, Ustinov, Branagh, Malkovich...left standing at the post.

And the **James Herriot** 'Vet' series.

And someone who isn't so well known but was a visceral writer and essayist: **Christopher Hitchens.** *Love, Poverty, War* and *God is not Great,* which mordantly slice open and leave in tatters the thrall all these tropes which hypnotise the world today.

And then, the old movies, happily found on YouTube:

Becket, with a petulantly electrifying Peter O'Toole as Henry II, and Richard Burton's Becket played with gravitas as a perfect foil;

The Lion in Winter, ditto and Katharine Hepburn, who won an Oscar for her role as Eleanor of Aquitaine;

Ryan's Daughter, one of David Lean's relatively unsung masterpieces;

1984, the seminal Orwellian dystopian prescient truth, with Burton and William Hurt showing us glimpses of the precipices on the brink of which we stand today in Bharatvarsh;

Julius Caesar, with the incomparable Marlon Brando as Mark Antony;

Sleuth, with Olivier and Caine in perfect tandem;

Henry V, with Olivier's Agincourt speech still ringing in my ears;

Finally, the old music. My time music of the 1950s and 60s. Music that is music and has withstood the barbed whips of rap and Indipop and nonsense lyrics (euphemism).

There is so much of it I could write about: The Moody Blues, The Beatles, The Stones, Jethro Tull, CSNY, Winwood, Alan Parsons, Mike Oldfield, Cream, Talat, Hemant Kumar, Manna Dey, Mukesh, Suraiya, Geeta Dutt, Mubarak Begum et al, all inimitable and who have stood steadfastly by me these past weeks.

But my abiding leading light was and is Jim Morrison of The Doors. The nonpareil Morrison in every sense of the word. Died young at the age of 27 (like his brilliant contemporaries whose names also started with 'J' – Janis Joplin and Jimi Hendrix), and left not just his music but his distinctive brand of unfettered poetry that was and is unparalleled for a rock musician, an oeuvre that deserves to be in any contemporary pantheon. I have a book of his musical poetry in his original hand. It is my musical Bible.

He was the quintessential Rider on the Storm.

He wrote, 'When the music's over, turn out the light'.

That is the only true philosophy of life. Know when to go, and how to go.

I could carry on.

But I won't.

Suffice to say, the dictum below is perhaps closer to our realities:

> *'Why didn't I learn to treat everything like it was the last time. My greatest regret was how much I believed in the future.'*
>
> —JONATHAN SAFRAN FOER,
> *Extremely Loud & Incredibly Close*

And finally, Doris Day might well have sung this instead in 2020:

> *'Que sera sera*
> *Whatever will be, will be,*
> *The future's not ours to see*
> *El pasado me pertenece (But the past belongs to me)'.*

One Day in the Life of a Miracle

Randhir Khare

I sit here, among potted plants, flowering creepers and fruiting shrubs, watching pariah kites wheel lazily in great circles, catching and flowing with the thermals, swooping then rising, high above pyramids of egrets gliding in from the river. The late afternoon is suspended in birdcalls and a low wind humming through the trellises of the garden fence.

My life until now was crowded out with living, 5 am to 11.45 pm and hurtling towards seventy. Thinking, feeling, writing, drawing, teaching, chasing purpose after purpose. Then suddenly the guillotine. The muscles and nerves of time sliced. Alive but limp. Unmoving. The city of Pune numbed, cut adrift, floating.

I have experienced times like this before... Bangladesh, the eerie calm before the bombers came in, Jalandhar before a terrorist attack, New Delhi before a lynching mob burst onto the street in front of AIIMS, the sudden deathly silence before the earth tore open Kutch. But this is different. I sit here and wait, in isolation, whilst all around me are other isolated human beings, waiting, whilst somewhere ambulances wail like hungry street dogs at night, and police megaphones bark orders.

I don't watch television, I don't read the news on my smart phone. I let the world take care of itself. I allow myself the long-earned luxury of savouring whatever breathing moments of my life remain. Yes, it is true what the Czech poet Vladimir Holan wrote in his poem 'Horoscope'...

'We understand simplicity only when the heart breaks,
And we are suddenly ourselves, alone and fateless.'

Yesterday does not matter, neither does tomorrow. All that really matters is the miracle of each living, breathing moment. And as Andre Gide asks, 'Don't you understand that the moment would not take on such incomparable vividness, if it were not thrown up...on the dark background of death?'

This morning, I gave myself to the pleasures of the senses as I set off on an early morning walk in the common spaces of our housing society, lined by numerous trees. Two entwined *neems* are there, alive with birds and insects. I ran my fingers over their trunks with affection, a twenty-year-old relationship in flower. I had planted them two decades ago and now they lean protectively towards my studio balcony. Beside them stands a raintree with its immense dome of green rustling with parakeets, minivets and passing feathered migrants who drift from tree to tree and shrub to shrub.

My dog, Tara, wasn't in the mood to mark her territory or run down cats. At nine, she's philosophical and calm, sniffs in the morning air, rolls on the grass then flattens back both her ears and smiles as if to say, 'it's time to head home for the morning slice of melon.' We relished it as we've done each moment of the day.

And now, the calm within expands and gives me space to lounge and read and I revisit books that I once loved and then abandoned. Each of them offer their own special fragrances and flavours. The woodiness of Walden, the fleshy otherness of E. E. Cumming's poems, the wine of Akhmatova's verse, wild orange rinds of Lorca's words, Neruda's sea drenched songs...I read them aloud. That disturbs Tara who looks around the studio for listeners, not finding them—she settles down at my feet and falls asleep, l am alone.

Alone at dusk, I stand at my studio's balcony and look up at the raintree bathed in the evening light—honey dripping from its leaves, bathing the backs of orioles, then falling drop by drop on the blossom-strewn earth below. Around me, everywhere, the city shuffles inwards, to feed and sleep, leaving me alone and undisturbed.

I cook a soup of celery, carrots, peas, onions and mushrooms, finely chopped and left to mingle the juices until the flavours of each blend into a whole. And as the whole turns and tumbles, bubbles, churns, I add fresh ginger chips and salt and peppercorns and basil, a spoon of barley flour. And then I watch it thicken slowly till it just about slides off the ladle. I dip in chunks of crusty bread and eat.

I am still alive, I know. The soup says so, the bread turns inside, settles and swells. I am wholly bread, late evening's bread of solitude, Time's bread…pushed and tongued, softened, dissolved.

A wind blows in the dark that watches me curiously as I, alone, sip after-dinner coffee and then pace my studio reciting Dylan Thomas' 'Fern Hill'…about the owls bearing the farm away and 'nightjars flying with the ricks' and horses 'flashing into the dark'.

Yes, it is time. Time for me to sit down and write poems that no one will read, draw pictures that will never hang on walls, write stories of forgotten times when there was love and hope and dreams that all came true. But then, isn't THIS why we write and draw? So that the moment has meaning? So that we liberate ourselves from our loves, our certainties, our hopes, our fears? So that we are finally free to create another reality? So that we can go beyond ourselves?

This is the moment when I lie down and wait to sleep, and I can't tell if I'm awake or I'm asleep. I levitate between the two. Rising from one and slipping into another. Am I afraid to close my eyes lest that's the last? I shake myself awake and like a waking dreamer turn in, listening to my body speak. It is a miracle that I'm alive and lying here and breathing.

I remember reciting the poems of the Czech poet Antonin Bartusek, standing on Charles Bridge in Prague, on the eve of the Velvet Revolution…lines of one of those poems rise to receive me as I fall asleep,

'At a time of such uncertain certainties
Such certain uncertainties –
It's dark in this room.'

I turn an empty glass face down beside my bed. This moment's passed.

A Lockdown Violation

Deepak Sanan

It has been a colder and wetter April than any I can remember in my decades of living in the hills. The pandemic has dampened more than just the spirits and the gloom of the lockdown has pervaded the weather. One Wednesday showed up in the forecast as a glorious sunny oasis in the midst of a daily dose of thunderstorms stretching on either side of the week. The day seemed tailor-made for a longer walk than the weather had allowed for a long time. Shalli peak, towering across our valley, beckoned. We packed lunch and coffee for a whole day out.

The closest starting point for the walk to the temple on Shalli peak is through a small forest clearing above the village of Khatnol. We drove through the deserted lockdown roads to reach there in a little over an hour.

The fine stands of deodar and blue pine, interspersed with cypress in the moist folds of the mountain, cast their shadows across glades carpeted with the freshness of soft green grass. There was a sparkle to the day and a spring in our step. We ascended to the top in better time than I had managed to do in all my years of visiting Shalli. Distant clouds marred a clear view of the snow peaks and perhaps foretold the ominous end to what had begun as a perfect day.

We reached our car to find the police, the press and a posse of locals awaiting our return. We had apparently violated lockdown rules in choosing to trek up to Shalli! Many hours of drama followed. We finally returned home after being booked under sections of the Indian Penal Code and the National Disaster Management Act for flouting official directions and causing the spread of the dreaded Coronavirus. For two days, the incident followed me in newspaper reports. Compared to most alleged violators of lockdown rules, I stood out as somewhat important, even though retired and certainly not in a position to cause trouble unlike the ruling party functionaries or serving officers!

My first thoughts were to understand the reasons behind the locals taking such an exception to our innocent excursion. We had met two other groups on the peak. They had climbed up by routes other than the one we had chosen. It appeared that only the denizens of Khatnol had taken such a strong umbrage to temple visits during the lockdown. Khatnol was in ferment over an incident involving a village girl studying in Chandigarh and wanting to return home. She had been stopped and placed in quarantine for fourteen days in the adjoining district of Solan. This was an affirmation, not only of the deadliness of the disease but of the fact that it could be carried by anyone coming from outside. Both our vehicle and our aspect, marked us as outsiders, deserving suspicion.

Finally, we had obviously upset egos by ignoring a random local telling us that the route to the temple was closed.

Underlying these immediate factors was a darker, more frightening scenario. The Coronavirus was being seen as a disease that rivalled the horror of the Bubonic Plague, during the Middle Ages. These droplets of death could be exhaled by even hale and hearty outsiders capable of climbing steep forest paths up to an elevation of almost 3,000 metres. And the noxious virus could linger and travel down from the forests to infect the village located far below! How had this fear psychosis reached such a pitch? Living in my isolated village home, I had somehow been oblivious to the manner in which official strategy and messaging had creating this situation.

A total lockdown, more severe than any in the world, almost complete cessation of business and movement and an injunction to stay indoors; a declaration of curfew implemented with utmost rigour by the coercive machinery of the state. From the moment the word lockdown had been added to our vocabulary, the messages were not so much about explaining the nature of the disease and the attendant risk, as castigating every incident of a positive case, as a calamity. The media has joined the frenzy. The entire focus is not so much on flattening the infection curve, as on somehow eliminating a scourge. An official colour coding of states and districts to represent their status as freedom from cases, has only added to the desire to somehow get rid of the disease. The attendant threat that the discovery of cases will be seen as a need for an area to revert to a more strictly-policed status reinforces this overwhelming objective. It is hardly surprising then that the fear and stigma, which touches even our loved ones, has quickly become the norm amongst people at large. That the lockdown was about flattening the curve, gaining time for the health system to be ready for an onslaught of cases, is implicitly jettisoned. Somewhere the wisdom, that all past pandemic-causing viruses had only attenuated through herd immunity, lies forgotten.

Much has already been written about the response of populist, right-wing leadership to the COVID-19 crisis across the world. The specifics of the Indian situation and why this lockdown and its attendant consequences suit the objectives of our rulers, have also received attention from a number of commentators. But what enables a popular buy into becoming a strategy that imposes mass suffering and is propagated by a regime with a history of lying? Why do lack of evidence of any great loss and an alternative, less onerous strategies find few takers? The desire to believe in the leadership in the face of an unforeseen threat is palpable. It is further fuelled by the predominant worldwide narrative that continues to emphasise that the disease has immensely frightening possibilities even though the horrifying projections of initial models have been belied, especially in countries like India.

Two interesting instances highlight this anomalous reality. One is about face masks. Despite lack of convincing scientific support for widespread use of face masks by the public, it is being prescribed and enforced across the world and has become the most visible symbol of the fight against the disease. The second relates to fatalities that can be ascribed to COVID-19. It is widely accepted that COVID-19 poses the greatest threat to persons with co-morbidity and age against them. On the one hand there is a debate on whether fatalities with co-morbidity should be reported as only COVID-19 related deaths. On the other hand, there is a viewpoint that even deaths from other causes (even without contracting COVID-19), that occur due to failure to receive medical attention because most facilities have been co-opted to serve COVID-19 possibilities (and are at least partially unused), should be chalked up against COVID-19!

What does all this portend for the Indian response to the COVID-19 crisis going forward?

A retreat from the course already charted requires the kind of statesmanship few countries are blessed with today. It needs a transparent sharing of available evidence and the possible options, an ability to take people into confidence and the humility to admit to the imponderables. In any case, the current approach of stamping out the disease with lockdown has too much going for it. The approach fits in well with the fear psychosis already created amongst the public. It furthers the image of the strong leader taking decisive action to squash the enemy every time it rears its head. It keeps the bureaucracy and coercive apparatus wonderfully focused on a single objective. Along the way it is aiding in the curbing of both dissent and recalcitrant voices from the states. We seem destined to a one step forward and two back approach. A constant process of crackdown with every new case which results in the creation and recreation of containment zones.

This means that in the foreseeable future, we are embarked on a downward spiral in terms of economic activity and livelihoods, since the disease will continue to make an appearance. Will this be sustainable for India? Many would like an upsurge, an Indian version of the Arab Spring. However, the portents hardly look promising for such an occurrence. The ruling dispensation certainly thinks they will weather the difficulties. Mass starvation will be avoided with the distribution of food grains that are in the process of being dispatched to all corners of the country. For the rest, the oft-quoted fatalism of the Indian masses will see them accept their lot. The blame will be attached to divine visitation rather than to any mishandling by the powers that be. I have sometimes laughingly spoken of a future for India in the North Korea mould. If this comes to pass then it may not seem so far-fetched to imagine a supreme leader, who can do no wrong, impoverished masses thankful to be allowed to exist and all worthwhile dissent, either incarcerated or in exile.

The Forgotten

Beetashok Chatterjee

We are in the third month of lockdown as I write this. The outlook is gloomy, resentment is growing, tempers are fraying and even the simple everyday routines of our lives—the 'old normal' lives we knew—seem like bliss. Unattainable. Who would have imagined that having brunch with a friend at a café would seem so heavenly that one could swoon at the thought? How about an outing to the beach to walk on soft sand, or splash in the Club pool with one's kids? I could go on and on about the simple pleasures of life. There is now a sense of foreboding, a feeling of isolation and uncertainty—wondering when this nightmare will end. Or if it will consume us before that.

Tough times indeed. Look at the numbers, changing by the minute. More than 7,000 dead in India at the time of writing; in the US, over 110,000! More than 400,000 dead worldwide. Scary. And none of the doctors and scientists have a clue yet as to how to fight it. A hundred theories, a thousand opinions...but no solution in sight.

We are living through a significant phase in history, come to think of it. Without trying to sound too dramatic, let us hope we're around to tell our grandchildren that we lived through the *Coronavirus of 2020*.

While we justifiably feel sorry for ourselves for having to suffer for something which is no fault of ours, have we ever wondered what life is like on the high seas in these turbulent times? On board the 50,000 odd merchant and some of the 4,000 odd naval vessels plying the oceans? On the many offshore oil rigs and platforms dotted across the globe located in deep seas? On the hundreds of ocean-going supply and salvage vessels currently at sea? How are the sailors on board these coping? I ask this because I am a seaman. I have been one for more than forty years, the last thirty or so as a merchant ship's Captain. Let me try and describe life at sea nowadays to you.

We all know what it is like to be in lockdown. We already have first-hand experience of this, correct?

Now take away all land from this equation and replace it with water. Take away all the roads, the parks, the trees and the sound of birds and pets. Let there be just water, water everywhere—as far as the eye can see. Nothing else on the horizon.

Next, take away doctors and nurses. (There may be doctors on board some naval ships, but there certainly aren't any on the others.) Then, take away family and friends—spouse, sons, daughters and buddies. Not enough? Take away television—news channels, entertainment, Netflix, Amazon Prime... Still not enough? Take away the Internet and social media. Leave behind just some WhatsApp messaging.

Now start adding. Add taking body temperatures twice a day, wearing face masks every time you step out of your cabin to go on duty, meetings or meals, casting a terrified glance at any shipmate who coughs or sneezes, knowing there is no medical help to be found. Add mental health issues—suicidal thoughts—that are bound to arise because of the isolation and the stress. Add working seven days a week, rain or shine, not knowing when they'll get to go home. Add living under a constant fear of infection from visitors in port.

Welcome to a day in the life of a seafarer. Leaving aside the body temperatures and the masks, this is a **normal** day for him/her. That is, when the rest of the world is **not** on lockdown and going about its daily business.

Behind the scenes, away from the front ranks of the COVID warriors (the doctors, nurses, the police); behind even the second ranks of the delivery boys, (the *kirana* shop owners, the garbage collectors and all those still trying to keep things running) are the seamen going about their duties quietly, transporting millions of tons of cargo across thousands of miles across the oceans. There they are on the high seas, locked down in floating prisons, at the mercy of Mother Nature and pirates active at various hotspots globally, forgotten and ignored by the rest of the world. They are trying to keep economies of nations alive, the wheels of trade running. Because there is no substitute for shipping.

Alas, they are never given the importance they are due. They are the forgotten tribe of warriors that nobody thinks about. They do not carry the glamour associated with airline personnel—no steely gaze under peak caps while walking briskly to the boarding gates, followed by a bevy of uniformed beauties struggling in their high heels to catch up. You may have passed a scruffy lot at airports though, during your travels—looking lost and out of place—seamen have the knack of looking out of place **anywhere** when not on board a ship at sea or in port.

Well, no more airports for them in the near future, I'm afraid. Seafarers across the world serving on ships currently have been told by their employers to forget about going home till this is over, as all international passenger flights are down and airports all over the world are closed. Shipping is seen as a non-essential activity. But is it? Should they not be allowed to travel by air to join ships where required and earn their livelihood, and to be allowed to go home at the end of their tour of duty? It will be a while before those at sea can be with their families again.

So let us spare a thought for the seafarers worldwide quietly performing an important service, and include them in our prayers. They deserve our support.

Let us not forget to remember The Forgotten.

Disquietude in Isolation

Jayshree Misra Tripathi

I smiled.

The day the fourteen-hour curfew was announced in Delhi. No, it was not malicious in intent, rather in amusement, with the thought of all the serials and films I would binge-watch. I still yearn to see all the Hindi films I had missed during my husband's overseas postings, over thirty years' worth!

My smile wavered when the 'lockdown' was declared a few days later for three weeks to ensure our safety, as the COVID-19 virus held the world in its thrall, with the fear of imminent death. Staggering daily figures of infections worldwide were alarming. Especially, the notable deaths initially in Europe.

I had asked my part-time helper to stay at home and sent her off with advance pay and supplies before the curfew was announced. I had felt something was not quite right since the first case had been detected in Kerala at the end of January. Household chores kicked in, leaving me weary at the end of the day. I set myself a flexible routine.

My smile faltered when this 'lockdown' was extended for another three weeks.

I hesitate to smile today, the third of May, as the 'lockdown' has been further extended by two weeks, with just a few restrictions lifted.

Yet, I had smiled at first, six weeks ago, at the thought of being isolated in my rented flat, socially distant from the neighbours till the air cleared…all I could think of was how I had once lived in semi-isolation over twenty-odd years ago, due to a political crisis. There was a shortage of petrol, so I was basically confined to my residence, far away from the city-centre where the mission was located, as was our son's school. Local transport was unsafe for foreigners during that time and taxis too, so I stayed still, at the residence, awaiting my family's return each day, often after fourteen hours. They would leave at six o'clock in the morning to avoid the traffic snarls and our son had to stay back at the mission until they could return. There was no curfew, no 'lockdown'—the agitations for political reform had been peaceful. I was isolated by circumstances. The turmoil continued for almost four months. So yes, the term 'lockdown' did not faze me.

These past weeks have been strange, waking up to bright sunny mornings, blue skies, white fluffy clouds and birdsong. In Delhi! The silence is pleasantly disturbing, to say the least. I certainly do not miss the cacophony of screeching tyres, cars honking, sirens blaring as ambulances rushed by, motorbikes revving loudly, at odds with the tinkle of the cycle rickshaw-wallahs' bells—the electric rickshaws ply silently but honk too! I do not miss the sound of the sports instructor at the school across the street, bellowing commands for forty-five minutes Monday to Friday, to which all I could do was roll my eyeballs and sigh!

I have long missed the silence of true solitude that lifts the spirit and encourages reflection, retrospection and the continued quest for knowledge. I have wanted to read certain books that I have kept aside for too long, as life got in the way—yearning for such silence. Mainly *The Upanishads*, translated by Eknath Easwaran, to overcome the feeling that I am getting old and just do not know, truly, the philosophical issues that have been thought of, debated, sung then transcribed centuries ago. It always humbles me.

These past weeks, I began to realise how grateful I felt for the sense of some tranquillity around me, apart from the odd sensation of hearing a sudden honk or a distant bark. Why are the street dogs not barking? Are they happier too? I do hope so. And no, I am not upset with the parrots sharpening their beaks on the green netting of the balcony–it is going to cost me a bit to replace it, once things return to normal. Will things return to normal? Will normalcy be redefined? Will physical distancing be the new norm?

As I pace across the rooms of my flat, I ponder upon the fact that as an urban flat-dweller, I am not close to nature. There are moments when I close my eyes and feel the soft grass beneath my bare feet, on different patches of lawn, in different lands. Armed with renewed positivity, I go and water my potted green air-purifying plants. I talk to them, out loud. Soon I may forget the sound of my own voice! Next 'to do' is to call a friend, a different one each day. The evening is for my mother in a distant state in southern India and my sisters who live with her.

I have no idea why the smartphone heats up–I am not one for long phone conversations.

I fret about the uncertain future–*Que sera sera,* my 81-year-old mother sings–yet I am filled with dread and the pain of mere anticipation which is acute and real. Past events are dredged into my present, but I seek them not! Where are the golden epiphanies? I am apprehensive of the immediate future.

The silence is peaceful, though my tinnitus sounds are now to the fore, and yet the few three-wheelers chugging down the gully below, probably carrying food supplies, do not disturb me. My reverie is interrupted by a voice through a foghorn, cautioning us with *Savdhan, Savdhan* and some information–reminiscent of the loud songs of new films to be released in the local cinema halls, played through the lanes and by-lanes of my childhood.

As the days have turned to weeks, my sporadic smiles have turned rueful. I do miss the sounds of cheerful chatter as the children rushed out of the school gates, eager to get back home. I miss the tantalising aromas rising from the food-stalls below, across the school gates. I must confess I sniff now and then, to ensure that I have not lost my sense of smell, a symptom of the COVID-19 virus, and continue to pace across the flat, to stay healthy, glancing quickly away from the exercise-strider I ought to be using for twenty minutes daily.

My thoughts turn towards the sudden rains and hailstones that had lashed Delhi and the surrounding NCR, nine days prior to the curfew. Traffic ground to a halt. Streets were flooded. The Ides of March. Nature settling its debts. Not the exact connotation, but a close one.

Much We Have Learned

Dilip Bobb

In recent weeks, I have been at the receiving end of a phonedemic. I have started getting a flurry of video calls from people I haven't communicated with for decades. We lost touch after they all moved to different cities and continents. One is now in Melbourne, another in London, a third in Paris and one in Toronto. They are all under some stage of lockdown and I am guessing that the sense of isolation and the comparative loneliness has inspired a subliminal urge for companionship. Also, a need to reconnect with the past, perhaps as a reminder of what friendship and camaraderie really mean, something we have all lost out on in the mindless sprint on the treadmill of modern life. Apart from discovering how the ageing process has affected long-lost friends, that sense of reaching out and reconnecting is one positive outcome amid the daily deluge of disaster and darkness. Hopefully, it may be part of the recalibration of life's priorities we will all undergo once this COVID madness is behind us. What the outbreak and lockdown have done is to prompt all of us to look at our lives with a fresh perspective. There is much we have learned in this challenging, stressful situation—social responsibility, resilience, compassion and kindness, even the benefits of proper hygiene and how not to mess up a home haircut. With billions around the world in some kind of lockdown, this is the largest psychological experiment ever undertaken. Many will emerge mentally battered by the experience but equally, a number may emerge stronger and more resilient, and certainly with greater empathy and feelings for our fellow countrymen and women.

This pandemic has also bridged the divide between the rich and poor—everyone is equally vulnerable, a situation that has given rise to the oft-heard phrase: we are all in this together. Technology has been the greatest asset for us all in lockdown mode. Long-lost friends have started or joined new groups on social media, while WFH (Work from Home) is the signature acronym of these troubled times. On an intellectual level, it has provided an opportunity to read more books, perhaps ones we would never have had the time or inclination for earlier. Imagine the unexpected joy of hearing world famous opera singer Andrea Bocelli's *Music for Hope* concert echoing across a deserted church in Milan. Over 3.4 million viewers worldwide tuned in to his YouTube performance, the largest audience for a classical music event ever. I have also been privileged to conduct a virtual tour of the world's biggest galleries, including the famous paintings of the Louvre in Paris and the classic sculptures of the Vatican Museums, from the comfort of my couch. My hope is that once this is over, people will realise that they don't need to return to their earlier lives of excess and extravagance, of buying the latest gadgets and filling our closets with stuff we really didn't need. The lessons are obvious, and there to be learnt.

Sympathy for the Devil

Sumit Mullick

I have been held captive in my house in Mumbai for over two months now, with no end in sight. I am not sure of the number of days, as I have lost sense of time. It is pointless to keep track of the passing of days, as each new day is indistinguishable from the last. Basically, I just eat and sleep, wash my hands, and keep my mind as subdued and dormant as possible. An active, thinking mind would brood and worry and, probably, lose its balance as it tries to assimilate all the horrible news coming from everywhere. Mumbai is, after all, the Coronavirus epicentre of India. No, it is far better not to think.

I can do without thinking, but the human requirement for love remains constant. But what do I love in the age of the Coronavirus? I am past romantic love, but I used to love the daily routine of my life...going to office to do some meaningful, self-satisfying work, taking a stroll down Marine Drive in the evening, having a drink with some friends in a pub in Colaba, going for a movie, watching a concert. All that is gone now, and a vacuum has been created. But nature abhors a vacuum. The void must be filled. I must find something else to love. And, gradually, almost imperceptibly, the emptiness has been filled by my captor, my tormentor, the Coronavirus.

Since I now have unlimited time, I started reading up on what being a virus was all about. I read about how the viruses, and their cousins, the bacteria, had been attacking and decimating human populations throughout our history. There were a vast throng of them…the Hanta virus, the Bwamba virus, the Arena virus, the Ebola virus, Leprosy, Tuberculoid and Yaws bacteria, and many, many others. They were mighty legions, with sophisticated weaponry, constantly innovating and refining their strategies, overcoming or bypassing defences.

And they could really decimate populations. The Bubonic plague in the sixth century C.E, called the Plague of Justinian, after the Roman emperor, killed an estimated 25 to 50 million, which was a big chunk of the global population then. In the fourteenth century, another Bubonic plague wiped out one third of Europe's population. The Spanish Influenza of 1918 killed 50 million. And, of course, there was the constant flow of Tuberculosis, HIV, Dengue and Malaria fatalities.

We all admire power. My respect and admiration for the virus began to grow. And this was real power, used with coordination, precision and intelligence. Intelligence? Was the virus intelligent? There was something much deeper about these microorganisms. So, I read deeper. I read that the Earth was formed around 4.5 billion years ago. And the first life forms had emerged just 300 million years later. And these first life forms were the ancestors of the same microorganisms that had been attacking us in the past and are still attacking us now. The virus had an excellent pedigree and an impressive lineage.

I also discovered that the virus really had a remarkable intelligence. To take just one example, there is a virus called the Lancet Fluke virus which infects ants. But the ants are not the real target. Ants are merely couriers. The virus enters the brain of an ant and persuades it to climb to the tip of a blade of grass, and just hang there and never let go. Then the sheep comes and eats the top of the grass, along with the ant and the virus. And then the humans eat the sheep. And the virus does very well, thereafter, in its new and final home. My sense of awe for the intelligence and strategic thinking of the virus skyrocketed.

But why are the viruses making so much effort, expending so much of their time and energy in attacking us, humans? Don't they have better things to do? There was nothing in the books I read that could enlighten me on this point. For that I had to use my imagination and enter into the mind of a virus. And after some very focused concentration, I succeeded.

When in the mind of a virus, I could hear the viruses communicating with each other in the primordial language of the beginnings of life, in the chemical language of amino acids, in the script of DNA/RNA. It was beautiful in its clarity and depth of reasoning. Here, let me tell you what they said:

'Our job is to ensure that all species live in harmony with each other, and with the Earth. And that no species prospers to the point that it is a threat to others. The chain of life is very complex, and hence very fragile. It requires constant policing. Throughout the history of evolution, we had to intervene on many occasions, whenever any species had become too dominant. We had to become the instruments of disease, sickness and death—all essential tools for a healthy garden, as for a healthy planet. We kept populations in check. We ensured that life never outstripped the available resources of the planet. We ensured that all species had a fair chance at the game of life.'

This was terrible, I thought. The Gaia hypothesis was correct. The Earth was a living body, and the microorganisms were its antibodies, created for the protection of the Earth. Protection from us, humans, who were destroying the Earth. So, would these microorganisms have to destroy us? I continued listening in fascination and horror.

'We destroyed the dinosaurs, because they had become too dominant and were not allowing other species to develop. Then we allowed the Homo sapiens to develop. But they developed too well for their own good, or for the good of other species, and of the planet itself. This cannot continue. But we have not exterminated any species since the dinosaurs. Exterminating a species is never an easy decision. Though we have the power, do we have the right?'

I listened truly amazed. The viruses had a very deep sense of morality and fair play. They were distressed. The contemplation of extermination was painful to them. They were far more moralistic than us, for whom extermination has been a normalised routine through the course of numerous genocides. They then started looking for arguments to save, not to destroy.

'Instead of exterminating, we can greatly reduce the number of humans. We can reduce them to the population size that existed when the species first began to emerge. They will then be too few and no threat to others, or the planet…'

At that point, I could no longer listen to what the viruses were saying. Either they had become aware of my presence and had switched me off. Or my imagination had dried up. So, I am not aware of their final decision regarding us.

Anyway, now I understand who my captors are. They are powerful, while being noble, wise and moral. Even though they have imprisoned me in my house, with a death sentence hanging over me, they have filled a void. Love has found a way in. I am in love with my captors.

Squash Blossoms:
Goa Lockdown Diary

Amrita Narayanan

When the lockdown is called, my first thought is to get rice but nothing is open. Goa's three-day curfew overlapped with the lockdown, so we were unprepared, and it would be days till we would be able to get essentials. Luckily a friend, who owns a shop, is able to give me two kilos of rice: all she has. Others are not so lucky: within a few days it is clear that there is no state plan for food, groceries are closed, and my WhatsApp lists are buzzing with messages about food shares and trades.

One message catches my attention: *I have Cilantro, Basil, Bhindi, Tomatoes, Squash, Local Lime and Doodhi for anyone who wants*. It's from my partner. Over a year ago, he had told me about a community garden he was planning at our daughter's school. The children would work the farm along with parents who wanted to. I hadn't wanted anything to do with it: as much as I liked the idea of fresh vegetables, I cringed at the thought of weeding in the sun and wasn't ashamed to say so. I would have many opportunities to ruefully recall the ease of my opt-out during the lockdown. We ate almost entirely from that community garden for a week, as we waited for the state government to sort out the food crisis. They were leisurely in their efforts.

Of the many foods we no longer have, my daughters complain almost immediately about missing juice and sweet soft drinks. They harvest a local Goan lime from the community garden, fist-size, like the *Gondhoraj*, as much orange as lemon. It makes a vivid green basil-lime cooler, and the girls happily de-stem fresh basil daily thereafter in anticipation of this libation.

We rotate through the vegetables we have, trying different things. My favourite discovery is pan-fried squash blossoms: we dip the yellow and orange *Lowki (Doodhi)* and Zucchini flowers in a chickpea and rice batter folded with chopped basil and crushed garlic, and pan fry them. The girls shriek as the oil splutters, and we all agree that they are delicious and must be made immediately the next day. We do, not only because we loved them, but also because the garden yields fifteen squash blossoms every morning that must not be wasted.

Despite the delights of farm-to-table, it's hardly the kind of moment in which there is time or inclination to post photos of sumptuous food and piles of novels waiting to be read on social media. Replete as it might be with moments of satisfaction, the lockdown is incredibly tedious. Cooking, sweeping, mopping, laundry and doing dishes seem to eat away large chunks of the day. Zoom meetings devour the rest, and yet leaves still more day in which to fold laundry, check messages and organise.

Within a few days the WhatsApp list is buzzing with messages about organising food for the migrant workers. One group member collects money, another works out a deal with the owner of a big grocery who agrees to sell large volumes of rice, dal, sugar and tea, a third puts together volunteers for deliveries and packing, there are twelve on the team altogether. Everyone is a bit scared: rumour has it that the cops have been heckling and sometimes beating people for curfew violations, even those in search of scarce food. I bite my tongue when P leaves with the truck that he generally uses for the community garden. He is gone for six hours: they have to dodge police, and food distribution takes longer when you are maintaining the 1.2 metre social distance. My girls and I make rag dolls and listen to Raffi Cavoukian's version of *Down by the Bay* over and over at the demand of the younger one. I am relieved as they dance around, happy to have a few minutes of reprieve from other realities.

Now that it has become clear that we can feed ourselves—and some others—from the garden vegetables, P is spending the early mornings there, and late evenings on the migrant food deliveries. During daytime I see patients via Zoom while he takes the kids. The warm, sometimes noble, feeling that accrues from helping other people does not spare us from the relentlessness of each other. There is a predictable pattern to the day, much like there was before the lockdown, but it involves only four three-dimensional human beings. Travel and excursions outside the home, including school for the children, usually provides the sponsorship for our family harmony. With these exits closed, we find ourselves frayed faster than usual.

Time loops, the days are slower and less eventful, an odd foil to the literally viral general anxiety and alarm. I miss transitions: the moment of entering the house after work, not knowing whether the children will be home or out playing; the whirl of goodbye kisses and lunchbox reminders before the morning carpool horn sounds; the delicious quiet after the children leave; the lingering in front of the closet to choose a sari trying to remember where all I will go that day; planning what to do over the weekend; waiting for a haircut; perhaps even the dratted doorbell whose existence I have cursed many a time.

Minus these inflection points, entries and exits, the lockdown stage set is oddly static. While the news is full of sorrow at the mounting losses and panic at what could be a potential impending crisis, the days stick together without separation, punctuated by WhatsApp forwards and memes, fingers traversing the screen in an unsatisfying desultory way.

When I made the *Doodhi* blossom fritters two days ago I swapped the basil in the batter for *chaat masala*, chopped onion and cilantro. My youngest was not fooled. 'This again?' she wailed. 'Amma has made it Indian style,' her sister explains, stifling laughter, 'at other times it was Italian style, tomorrow Amma will make it uhhh Antartican style.' Her sister whispers something, pokes her indignantly and they collapse in giggles.

I open my phone to show them photos of their own and their friends' parents packing and distributing food packets. They must know I feel, how lucky we are to have food at all. Then I realise that the desire to shake them out of giggles into care and concern, has less to do with their needs than with mine. I was motivated by the uneasy memory of my former carefree unconcerned self, the one who thought she didn't need to put her sweat into a kitchen garden, happy to be able to afford store-bought organic vegetables, the former self to whom it would not occur to panic-buy, who had not imagined that her government would leave no provision for food supply. For that naive self, already ill in the aftermath of the CAA, the Corona pestilence has closed a door permanently: no return to solipsism in the present, deathly interconnected, world disorder.

The Unsung Journalists

Lalita Panicker

The late, great journalist Marie Colvin once said, 'Bravery is not being afraid to be afraid.' Brave beyond all limits, she went where the story was–from the killing fields of Sri Lanka where she lost an eye when she was struck by a blast from a rocket-propelled grenade to finally, the vicious battlegrounds of Syria, where she was killed in a rocket attack in Baba Amr, striving to the very last to make the voice of the voiceless victims of violence heard. We know of her, have read books on her, seen documentaries about her extraordinary life and commitment to reporting.

As we face an insidious virus today, health workers are getting their place in the sun, something they should have got long ago. We honour them and recognise their role in making a difference between life and death for millions. I write this from a position of privilege; I am an opinion writer, I can insulate myself and frame analytical pieces based on news. I can go out and meet people when I choose to, listen to their opinions if I want to enrich my knowledge or go out in the field to try and bring a touch of the human element into my analysis.

But who gets us the news? Day after day, it is the unsung reporter, photographer or stringer who goes out into the field, armed with nothing more than rudimentary protection to bring us the stories of this pandemic.

A journalist friend of mine, in charge of a large posse of reporters, told me about her mental stress and fear when she had to send her reporters out into the field. They have to traverse the narrow alleys of urban slums, the overcrowded wards of hospitals, enter tiny ramshackle dwellings, walk on the highways where desperate people, bereft of work and seemingly of hope, trudge to try and get back to their homes. These newspersons have to return to their homes and insulate their families from their presence lest they are carrying the dangerous virus back with them, picked up in the course of work. My friend was filled with trepidation, what if one of her staff caught the virus? Would she also not be responsible, as much as the organisation for which they all worked? Yet, she spoke of the extraordinary willingness of her staff to try and bring back the best stories, both heart-rending and elevating, of how people are dealing with the crisis.

When you wake up every morning, you reach for your newspaper, however truncated it is today. Or you switch on the news or go online to learn of what new invidious ways the virus is affecting our lives. Behind each story you read, each bit of information you digest, every image you see, a reporter, a photographer, even star journalists have gone out into what is now being described as the battleground to bring you those. Many of them are people who are not in the public consciousness, they are not the high decibel media demagogues who rail at us each evening from the comfort of their studios. But while our health workers deserve three cheers for their valiant contributions, surely the media persons out in the field deserve at least two.

I have been out there myself in my salad days and I know how difficult it actually is to bring you the news. For a start, unless you are a brand, a big enough name or from a big enough media outfit, you simply don't have access to many news sources. You have very little by way of resources. In one organisation I worked for, one of the richest in India, maybe the world, a reporter covering an ongoing violent incident in another state was astounded when the management head told him to take a bus to the location to save money knowing full well that time was of the essence. In the *mofussil* towns of India, women reporters have harrowing tales of being given accommodation in somewhat shady hotels on account of their measly budget. Many, especially women, face many hurdles traversing rural areas even today when things have improved vastly in the media. Yet, some of the most magnificent stories, some of which have changed the course of politics, of society, of development and, yes, humanity, have come from the inimitable commitment and dedication of these journalists.

Today, as I write, several reporters in television channels and the print media have contracted the virus. No one has clapped for them, banged thalis or shown any other signs of solidarity. It is our job, you might say, so get on with it and stop seeking affirmation and applause. Yet, the millions of words and images that stream into our homes through the media every day, every hour, every minute carry with them a certain authority. Is this public trust misused? Yes, it is through fake news on social media and shoddy reporting. But still, the overwhelming information flow is based on hard work, unseen research, careful fact checking and sparkling writing.

Not to diminish the threat from the Coronavirus, reporters, photographers and others out in the field in India constantly face dangers in covering cataclysmic events. Riots, natural disasters, epidemics, seasonal diseases, terrorism are just some of them. They have to bear witness to dreadful images of the sick and dying, of murderous mobs, of victims of wasting diseases, of inhuman living conditions, of starvation and death, of violence and the silence of graveyards. There are no counsellors to help them process these images, to deal with the horrors which will never reach your homes through the media because they would be too upsetting to you, and rightly so.

I am sure you all have seen or read about the infamous photo of a vulture edging close to a dying child trying to reach a feeding centre in Sudan taken by legendary photographer Kevin Carter in 1993. He won a Pulitzer prize for it in 1994 and four months later took his own life. The horror of what he had seen, perhaps his inability to help the child, or his guilt over gaining accolades from death and misery was too much. This is an extreme case, but just to emphasise that it is not easy to be up close and personal to death and disease as thousands of reporters and other newspersons are doing today facing down the Coronavirus.

A Providential Life with the Coronavirus

Anita Anand

In many ways, providence had prepared me for COVID-19.

In September 2018, on the second day of my art exhibition for which I had been preparing for months, I fell and broke the tibia in my right leg in three places. Post-surgery, with a rod and screws in the leg, I was homebound for close to six months, with monthly visits to the doctor for a check-up and some social visits around that. It was a wheelchair existence, somewhat exacerbated by the fact that I chose to be on the second floor of my home. Negotiating the stairs (especially while ascending) was a challenge.

In February 2019, the orthopaedic surgeon suggested that I may need a graft, as the break just below my knee was not fusing as it should have. I was hesitant, not wanting another surgery, and asked that we give more time for the bone to fuse. In subsequent visits and X-rays there was some progress and the graft discussion, happily, was laid to rest. However, a CT scan in mid-October indicated that a graft was necessary.

My son was to be married at the end of November. The doctor assured me I would stand that day, *sans* wheelchair, walker or stick. I smiled but deep down I knew this was not going to happen. The surgery was done. Predictably, I was in a wheelchair during my son's wedding and later I even took a trip to southern India with my close friends who had come from outside India. Everything on a wheelchair. I had told myself it did not matter.

I was conscious and somewhat uncomfortable about the inconvenience I was causing those assisting me with my immobility. But, the generosity and kindness of everyone was overwhelming and heart-warming.

Like before, a long period of recovery from the surgery loomed ahead. But I was prepared and accepted it. I was fortunate that both the times I was immobile during winter so I could enjoy the terrace garden and appreciate it through the glass doors and sit in the sun. My son and his wife came to live with us for a few months and that brought about some changes in the household. Welcome changes.

The 2018 fall was not my first. In December 1999, the year I had turned fifty, I had fallen down and broken the fibula in the same leg in Chiang Mai, in Thailand. I had a surgery and a rod and screws were inserted. When I came back to Delhi where I live, I could not function. Not a crutches person, I found it hard to go around, sleep, move or be comfortable.

After the initial period of frustration and despair, I learned to cope with my immobility. Wheelchair bound for months, I went out with the assistance of my husband, with the only major challenge of not being able to access toilets. I cancelled most of my professional and social life for six months. It was my last year of full-time work. I was anxious about the future; about disengaging from my profession; yet staying engaged and making a living. What would fill my hours?

Serendipitously, many things came into my life. A book contract and an opportunity to be involved in organising a global conference on 'Mountain Women in Nepal'. Things were looking up.

It's not like I was not used to illness. A lifelong asthmatic, I had struggled with the handicaps of the disease. The advent of inhalers and antihistamines has helped me manage my asthma. With each subsequent surgery since 1999—five in all, including two eye surgeries for a detached retina—I had learnt what it meant to be incapacitated and to not take my health for granted.

After retirement from full-time work, I was nudged towards a more spiritual life. I began to work more with my hands; I began painting, cooking and baking. I studied hypnotherapy and started a practice with three other women. By a stroke of luck, I was asked to travel to Afghanistan in 2004. It was my first time in a post-conflict country. I returned several times, developing a closeness to the country, with the people and experiencing the challenges posed in building a nation.

In 2008, I was fortunate to attend a retreat in Delhi led by the Zen Buddhist monk and teacher, Thich Nhat Hanh. I was struck by his teachings and the simplicity of the recommended practice of mindfulness—in which we do everything we do, mindfully. I began practising with a Sangha, a community of practitioners, and found a sense of peace and calm, which I had not experienced before. Mindfulness asks that we live in the moment, not in the past which has gone or the future which is unknown. We only have the present.

So, when COVID-19 arrived, I was already on a kind of lockdown, a physical one—and had been for twelve of the last eighteen months. My husband and I have been working from home since 2007. We chose to move outside the city and build a home in a quieter neighbourhood. As part of a privileged class and family, we opted to have a full-time helper and his family live with us, which has helped us cope with the day-to-day tasks at home, when the lockdown was announced. Other routine work such as car cleaning, ironing clothes, cleaning and gardening is done by part-time staff, who are staying in their homes now and we are in touch with them. We support the people living in the settlements around us however we can; we contribute to the local gurdwara and several NGOs who are helping those who have lost their livelihoods.

In March, a few weeks before the lockdown, I had started venturing out, cautiously, not taxing my healing leg. A friend asked me about my plans for the rest of the year. I laughed and said: No plans.

I am grateful that my life experiences and choices have allowed me to be prepared for COVID-19. I continue to paint, write, bake and tend to my garden. I meditate and am calm. I know COVID-19 too, will pass.

Corona-Rekha Wrap

Tuktuk Ghosh

When Prime Minister Narendra Modi drew the Corona-Rekha for his *'pyaare* 130 crore *deshvaasiyon'* in a televised nationwide address, effective 24 April 2020, in the uber-protective mode of Lakshman in the eponymous epic, *Ramayana*, many of us accepted the enforced *ghar-bandi* with remarkable resignation of what was by then a screaming inevitability. After all there could be no quibbles about the greater public good, as the clamour for it had been rising by the day, in particular from the medical fraternity. WHO had declared a pandemic and many countries had shuttered down as the only way of defending themselves from the insidious assault of a swiftly advancing invisible enemy.

Whether our government was adequately prepared for, arguably one of the most severe lockdowns globally, will endure as a favourite subject for unending discourses across many super moons. As a retired bureaucrat, this did not appear to me to have been the case. I found myself involuntarily whooshing around to figure out the why of it all. Obviously, the reasons had to do with the totally unprecedented, unimaginably colossal nature of the health emergency and the trademark stumbling-bumbling *andaaz* of *sarkari* functioning. A la the yet-to-be-understood *note-bandi* of 2016, there have been torrents of guidelines, advisories, clarifications, statements and retractions leaving the best and most adept dumbfounded.

However, I will reserve the venting of mega *angst* for some other, suitably appropriate platform even as I continue to wrestle with it unendingly and get knocked down unceremoniously in the challenging process ever so often.

To move to a more personal note, I must confess I experienced what was unfamiliar, mildly disturbing and a strange feeling in the Corona-Rekha Wrap, notwithstanding its stoic acceptance. The one that will haunt me is of being literally forced—absolutely contrary to my core persona—into conjuring up grim threats to basic wellness in just about any and everything, as also in everyone around and redesigning the most basic of responses with varying degrees of artifice. It has been the response to even something as mundane as an appreciative touch! The novel virus has made a harsh demand for PPE—personal protective equipment—not only in a physical sense, but also as a basic emotional one. Bizarre, at times, and hugely challenging, but there is no escaping compliance. The loss of wee bits and pieces of cherished sensibilities is unsettling, knowing that it will not be a temporary phase.

How much isolation and distance are feasible to create and maintain and at what cost, especially within the four walls of a shared living space I wonder! And I am talking of shared as in terms of decades! Being constantly on high alert to fend off real or imagined assaults, being suffused with suspicion, placing oneself above all else, are the unusual, yet supremely pragmatic prescriptions. The risk and unspeakable consequences of being careless, in a manner of speaking, are entirely yours. It almost feels like Humpty Dumpty's big fall, albeit in painful slow motion, with no end in sight, reaching out for fragile slivers of cautious hope and naïve prayers to escape the wrath of the most vile enemy of the moment.

It is almost impossible to put the overturned lifestyle into any reasonable, comprehensible context. This tough balancing act, on a continuously fraying tight rope, has admittedly proven to be daunting.

The info-rush on public health, medical science, technological innovations, governance policy patterns and all matters connected, that has come as an unavoidable add-on with the Corona-Rekha Wrap is, without exaggeration, tsunami-like in its force. What makes it hugely complicated is that there cannot be any serious fact checking on an ongoing basis. Be that as it may, I admit to the subtle fascination of a cognitive *terra incognita* where I find myself marooned, notwithstanding sharp tinges of the fearsome and morbid, of the fast morphing near-future and beyond.

There is this nugget that has cast its spell on me in that space. It does not matter whether it's simply make-belief as it sums up altered reality with amazing impact. The weight of a virus is about one millionth of a trillionth of a gram. With the number of cases worldwide crossing millions in the space of a few months, it is surprising to know that it has taken only over one gram of a virus to bring mankind to its knees. Is this brute power of nature unleashed in glorious ferocity or payback for its ruthless desecration?

Zooming back to the Corona-Rekha Wrap imperatives—Stay Home, Stay Safe—was the only option available to the nightmare of official highhandedness, roughly coated in a resuscitated century-old legislation, quarantine in a hellhole, no known available treatment and livid chaos in hospitals, desperately trying, without adequate infrastructure, to control the overwhelming catastrophe. These are the indisputable grisly home truths.

But when biggies and celebs made it sound greatly exciting and fun, as I believe they were cajoled into doing and also as it may have actually been for them, I couldn't help recoil many a time in agitated despair and frustration. The glib gloss stampeded with heart-rending images littered across all mediascapes of thousands, who had no home to retreat into and chill, who had just been abandoned to cruel fate. Unspeakable apathy, which we, the mainstreamed and comfortably off, had, in a sense, become unwitting parties to, burned a deep wound, which will perhaps not fully heal. Human misery, so callously dismissed, brought out deep visceral reactions which I am still trying hard to deal with.

Same for the upsurge of sheer loathing, stigmatisation, ostracism and hate that was on full public display towards the unfortunate victims of the virus, minority communities and professionals tasked to deal with it. The depths to which we can sink with effortless ease has been stunning to witness and acknowledge.

I realise it's an uncomfortable shade of dark that I am grappling with and the perspective lens could do with a positive reset.

This becomes all the more important when now we are told that the virus will be around forever and that the Corona-Rekha Wrap must be armoured with '*atmanirbharta*', while it mutates ominously and unpredictably.

So Now You Know

Supriya Newar

So now you know what is an enforced distance,
It's all I've known; my presence only met with resistance.

So now you know what it feels like to be caged,
I've lived it for years, all along held my enrage.

So now you know what it is like to lose a dream,
I gave mine up eons ago, each one went unseen.

So now you know the ennui of unending chores,
I've performed them silently, as you tallied bigger scores.

So now you know the low blow of uncertainty,
Rarely have I managed more than a word in the finality.

So now you know what it's like to not be in control,
I was expected to settle for less, to strengthen the whole.

So now you know what helplessness feels like,
While in chains of morality you've long had me tied.

So now you know the value of immunity,
For long I've endured your abuse, your impunity.

So now that you too know of a lockdown,
Will you reawaken?
Will we finally have a vaccine
To your mindset, to your discrimination?

Pause

Supriya Newar

Have you ever known a creature as strange as man,
Who always wants what he can't have, not happy with
what he can.

He has long discovered fire and rolled out the wheel,
He's made trillions of dollars and cut every possible deal.

He's split up an atom to create nuclear fission,
His stride knows no bounds, there's no end to his mission.

He's fought bad weather, high seas and the dark,
Seemingly conquering nature, emerging monarch.

In his own little trip, he's so ignorantly wound,
He forgets he's part of nature, it's not the other way
around.

But Mother Nature, as we call her, is both ageless and
wise,
She knows how and when to cut him to size!

She doesn't do much, just grants him his will,
Of time flying he complains, she brings it to a still.

He doesn't trust the other, or considers him too small,
She facilitates a distance and now there's a wall.

She'll repeat these lessons for as long as it takes to understand,
We're a speck of the whole, though we think ourselves grand.

That we can't endanger other life forms and continue to prevail,
That we too may get locked out and we may all ail.

That we're here to coexist, not to loot and conquer,
That the earth is our cradle, our only anchor.

It's time man's arrogance began to drop,
It's time man learnt, when it's time to stop!

Of Social Unavailability and Silver-lined Culinary Playbooks

Sushmita Bose

The eerie daytime stillness persisted for well over two months, punctuated by birdsongs and sounds of pressure cookers going off nearby. Like nights are punctuated by the swish of fans or the hum of air-conditioners when I get up for a drink of water...or when I am jolted back to wakefulness after a bad dream.

Hours, days, weeks and then months became blurs. After the initial burst of determination that I will keep track of time and be mindful, I was living in a surreal haze. I had lost count of clocks ticking, dates and days of weeks. But, yes, I'd occasionally remember to shake my wristwatch because I feared it may go into terminal shutdown lying on my bedside table at a time when time stood still.

The first couple of weeks, I was philosophical. There was food (Zomato, Swiggy and the friendly neighbourhood grocer—whose shop remained open since its services were deemed 'essential'—went about business as usual), entertainment (zeroed in on compelling shows on Netflix and Amazon Prime), and a comfortable state of living—aesthetically as well as experientially... It helped greatly I was in company—albeit sullen at times, since the lockdown, never mind candlelight vigils and clanging of utensils, was getting to everyone.

In the kick-off fortnight, I philosophised. Contemplated about localised living, whittling down wants and needs, doing away with luxuries, travelling virtually... mulled over the joys of tweezing eyebrows at home, of not having to worry about running out of a particular shade of lipstick, the wonders of #LockdownMemes, the wisdom of new webinar-based business models and so on.

But by the third week, I was in the grip of a mental health crisis. Not the shrink-seeking sort; it was about being hemmed in, gasket-like, by insulation. I'd become socially distant. For all my life, I've fancied myself to be a people's person. I like gabbing. The more nonsensical, the better. Therefore, my fondness for the phrase 'bonfire of inanities'.

As we veered into Lockdown 2.0, I started dreading gabbing. Okay, make that virtual gabbing, virtual socialising. I exited WhatsApp group chats where friends, locked down in various parts of the world, wanted to do Zoom calls (one was supposed to have been over a glass of wine). I was terrified of seeing sari and ingredient challenges on social media—those showcases of like-minded individuals in a favourite drape or holding out a dish made with, say, cinnamon powder—and logged out of Facebook when a friend tagged me. I changed my WhatsApp setting so my 'last seen' couldn't be seen by contacts. My phone remained in silent mode; whenever I got a missed call, I'd send a text message saying—lying—I'm in the middle of something, call you back later...and obviously didn't follow through.

If anyone were to ask me, what was the thing I hated most about the lockdown, I'd have to say a WhatsApp message called 'Hey, how are you doing?'—or any of its other manifestations. Since I didn't have an answer, here I'd plain speak and write back, 'I'm sick of people asking me that' along with a smiley. Most of my friends, to their credit, cottoned on.

Social media also proved to be a teaser platform of serials to 'binge on'. Everyone and his/her grandparents were overdosing on *Paatal Lok* or *After Life* or *Fauda*.

App-based OTT streaming channels have been part and parcel of our lives for a while now. But while during 'normal' times, there was a semblance of routine and its attendant narrowcasting, during lockdown the shows went on and on...and on.

After Life, for instance, was mind-numbingly good, but even before I'd savoured it and given it its due salute, I had wandered on—knowingly—to something else, something better (like *The English Game*), or worse (like *Manifest*). And in the ensuing cacophony of adapted screenplays and original ones, I was losing sight of everything...afterlife included.

I couldn't help but think back on those halcyon days when watching a show was an absolute treat, something that would stay with you for a week or a fortnight, and then get embedded in your mind like a sim card whose memory storage capacity never ran out.

At times, I'd run my fingers along the linear contours of my neglected DVD player and DVD box-sets, and promised I'll see more of them the moment I get back to conscious living...to put a cap on conspicuous consumption, to be grateful for lines of control.

But there was a silver-lined culinary playbook. Whenever I felt a need to be creative, I cooked. It was the best outlet for all my frozen energy. I remembered how I scoffed at someone in Hyderabad telling me—this was when I was physically there, months before I'd heard of a strain called COVID-19—the women in his family cooked from early morning till late evening. Over the lockdown, I discovered the joys in my kitchen kingdom, and I suddenly empathised with those Hyderabadi women.

Cooking was my only connect to the world outside because it balanced creativity with a method-bound timetable. There is a system, a timeline and you can't afford to be complacent (unless you want bad food). I now knew that potatoes get boiled to a single pressure cooker whistle. That how much of salt you need to put is a gut feel. That the good old mortar and pestle does almost everything a mixer-grinder does. That you need different knives for different operations—however sharp they may be. That Dalgona coffee can be as good as a Starbucks one—if you put your heart, and traction, into it. That you actually need to follow a timer when you knead flour for *poori*s.

Cooking (finally) managed to get the mush out of me in fits and starts. It softened me while I got the meat tender and the pasta *al dente*. The same friends I had tried dismissing when they wanted to meet online, messaged me endlessly when super cyclone *Amphan* hit Kolkata—they know that a significant chunk of my life, in the form of family, friends and emotions, continue to reside in that city—and connected the dots.

My abiding memory of the lockdown was emerging from the kitchen, washing my hands carefully—not because of Coronavirus, just to get the mutton rezala smell off—and going through my contact list. And calling or texting every single person who belonged to Kolkata, locked down as a storm raged and an insidious virus sneaked around.

Three Lockdown Lessons

Sohan Hatangadi

Hair-raising experiment

I fancy myself an efficiency expert and therefore, I started looking for ways to cut down every unnecessary task that I could. It was lockdown; I was not meeting anyone. When I did go out for some quick shopping, it was like a surgical strike, I covered half my face with a surgical mask and was in and out of the store in minutes. In one of these store visits, I discovered the cost of the Gillette Mach3 razor cartridges—'the best a man can get'—with 'stronger than steel blades', was a stupendous Rs. 130 per cartridge! I took my first major lockdown decision. I gave up shaving!

My facial hair grows at a slow pace. So, it took a while for the spiky little hair bits to start sprouting from my cheeks, chin and upper lip. Somehow, in a gravity-defying feat, the bristle all started growing perpendicular to my face, instead of downward. It looked menacing but I convinced myself that the follicles would soon settle down and flow smoothly over my cheeks, giving me a dignified statesmanlike look. As the days passed, every time I looked at myself in the mirror, I reminded me of what a 'boogie man' looked like, in those insensitive children's books. Then, my grey hair on my head started growing wild, and it turned out the barber shops were all closed. While I imagined smooth flowing locks, my facial hair looked like worn-out bottle brush. Then, it started itching! I imagined that some little creatures were making a colony in the beard. Every time I looked in the mirror, I suspected that I looked like a typical bum but kept hoping that those looking at me might find some redeeming features in my mug. All this time, I refused to video-chat with my grandson so as to not scare him for life.

My better half indulged me at first but when, push came to shave, she finally decided that enough was enough and asked me to pull myself together and remove the shrubbery from my face. She offered to help my transformation by clipping off the ends of the hair over my ears. So, one day I shaved off my beard but clung to my moustache. Meanwhile, Spacio, my saloon opened and I got a neat haircut. A few days later I removed that offensive strip of hair on my upper lip. Finally, I had become a clean-shaven gentleman. I could face my family and not scare my grandson. The lesson I learned was that lockdown or not, mask or not, growing a garden on the face is a challenge I shall not attempt ever again.

Webinarcism

I decided that we should make the best of lockdown by learning something interesting. Online seminars were being offered by many and they were all free. Now, I am no cheapskate but the word 'FREE!' makes me sit up and want to participate. The subjects had a nice intellectual sound to it. 'Deccan Legacy', 'Housing of migrant workers', 'Impact of COVID-19 on urban planning', 'Data Science and the role of technology', 'Localising volunteerism' and so on. So, I loaded up the Zoom app, plugged in my headphone and microphone, tested out the equipment and registered for every online seminar I could get on. I imagined that they would all be participative and that I could also pitch in my two paisa bit. But when I did log in, I discovered that there were several participants like me and they were all muted for video and audio.

While some of the meetings were quite interesting, others were an ordeal. Broadband connections would be lost, audio and video would vanish momentarily and PowerPoint presentations would mysteriously not show up on the screen. As this was a time when speakers started experimenting with the virtual meetings, there were many who were pregnant with knowledge of the subject but no clue on how to deliver the talk in an interesting way. We all know the famous formula $E=B^2$ which translates to *Expertise is proportionate to Boring Squared.*

On many occasions, as the speaker droned on, I was tempted to leave the virtual meeting, but the departure of a registered participant would show up on the app; therefore, I would just keep the app on and slink away to take a cat nap. Then, just before the meeting ended, I would come back and make a parting remark. After a few days my thirst for free knowledge on the internet subsided.

I decided that I was getting all the knowledge I needed from watching science fiction and crime movies on Netflix and the rest on National Geographic or Discovery. It was enough to satiate my locked-down brain with the nectar of knowledge. So, my second takeaway from the lockdown was that the thirst of knowledge could be avoided successfully with some discipline and innovation.

Overcoming the social distancing blues

Eventually not meeting friends for long periods becomes depressing. Especially when we have met face to face on weekends for decades, typically for an evening of celebratory beverage, discussing profound subjects like interplanetary space travel and the comparative taste of Godavari brown prawns and sea prawns. For some time, we spoke wistfully on the phone, then the possibility of seeing each other on the phone on WhatsApp video chat came up. We decided that we would have a virtual meeting, lift our glasses and say 'cheers!' to each other. The permissible group size was four and that was OK, because that was the number of eager drinking buddies I had at a time to participate in such virtual parties. Ah, the wonders of technology!

So, we filled our glasses, aimed our phones towards ourselves, making sure that our faces and the raised glasses were both in the frame and we yelled 'Cheers' in the most cheerful way. It was fun, and we got a kick out of it for a couple of weekends but then this 'cy-bar' business went out of style. We missed the real thing. To add to the dark mood, there was a cloud hanging over our liquor cabinets. Andhra Pradesh is going through the withdrawal symptoms at the moment. After the government took over the liquor business in preparation to prohibit the stuff, the lines outside liquor stores have been long, the price of liquor has gone through the roof, and one cannot buy a decent bottle of beer to help us survive the travails of summer.

They say that all good things will end. If that is true, then all shitty things must also come to an end. Sooner or later this pernicious virus will also stop troubling us. Life will go back to normal. We will shave and groom ourselves every day, we will attend seminars physically, shake hands and hug our friends. We will burn our masks and meet at each other's homes to play music, pour ourselves a chilled beverage and say 'Cheers! Cheers! Cheers!'

Itna Karo Na Mujhe Pyaar!

Pooja Poddar Marwah

In this #Quaratinemodeon lifestyle, one thing is for certain. Life goals are at their peak for everyone you know and perhaps, even the ones you don't. Everyone has their unique way of putting living into life. And of course, flaunting it as well. I admit, I am guilty as charged too.

It is scary out there and there is no denying it. The uncertainty that tomorrow will bring is not reserved for a special few but to humanity as a whole. Everyone is doing their bit to ensure the comfort and safety of the people that mean the most in their life and if today, you sit down and look around...you will realise that your own circle of life is right around you.

This is what you wake up for. This is what you work and strive hard for. This is the laughter that drives you. These are the tears that break you. In the end, when everything is taken away, these are the ones that will cherish you.

Over the past few weeks, I have been getting a lot of calls and messages, asking about my health. The parameters are all aligned, as they should be, as of the present moment and I greatly associate that with being a SPIRITual woman!

Walking with John, perhaps! Did I omit mentioning Walker?

If there is one thing I have learnt in the past few weeks, it is that life is meant to be lived. Someone will judge you and someone will not. Someone will love you and someone will not. So, I figured as most people my age do, that getting closer to the SPIRITual journey would give me the peace and dedication necessary to achieve my moksha. Now, please don't take it any other way than it is intended to be. But this is my guideline for attaining the highest form of freedom. It is believed that to reach this sacrosanct level, one must give up all desires and become SPIRITual so, I woke up one 'chilled Corona' morning and decided that this would be my awakening.

I set my alarm to a calm soothing tune and woke up to Shakira's *Waka Waka*. I didn't snooze the alarm nor did I crawl out of bed. Oh No! I jumped out and that too with a smile. After all, I can only spread happiness if I am happy.

The day went by with the mind buzzing with the morning tune. Work got done faster, chores even more so. Being a weekend, orange juice was naturally a healthy option. An extra special spiked shot of Vitamin C. After all, it creates antibodies and helps kickstart the immune system.

The day matured into an evening with a fuzzy head and a creative imagination. And, I refuse to divulge further on the latter words. But I am doing the best I can, to be a SPIRITual woman. After all, it is the eternal freedom I am seeking.

The Mr comes up to me and looks strangely. 'Are you feeling alright today, darling?' And I look at him, calm and composed, 'Yes of course, my dear. You always wanted me to be a SPIRITual woman, didn't you?'

He gave me the look that screamed INSANE but said nothing. I sat back on the rocking chair and had a heart-to-heart with the man... John Walker, I mean... Or do they still call him Johnny?

Given the current situation we are all faced with, a little bit of humour does no one any harm. Life is all about nurturing the right perspectives. In the toughest moments, it is in this mindset that some sail through and some don't. It is what it is and everyone is doing their best to make the most of this trying period.

I can't say for you but I sure am inspired to attain the freedom that comes with being SPIRITual.

Enough has been said of HER and enough is being done for HER. How about we sit out now and open a pint of Corona...just to tell HER that we are in high SPIRITS to overcome, all that SHE throws our way!!

In my defence, all I want to say is—*Itna karo na mujhe pyaar*!!

Liberation

Avijit Dutt

It was on 19 March, 12:30 pm that the call came in. 'Mitron…' threatened us in the evening. Definitely tough measures would be announced. We had to make our plans. Wuhan in China had closed down; America was being battered, as was Europe. Jokes about the Vodka Belt not being hit by the virus were still funny.

But what of the boys from my healthcare initiative working in the villages of UP? I was winding up a meeting in Greater Kailash, when news came of Section 144 being promulgated in UP. We conferred and decided that the boys were to leave behind the larger equipment in a hired office in the village and return, before the PM's speech, to Delhi. I was sure we were heading into a lockdown, but mistakenly believed that it would be for a few days. So, with all assets (human) back in Delhi, I was relieved. Temporarily.

Then began the wait. First the day long 'Janta Curfew' became the lesser benign lockdown, thrust from the top with low tolerance. All transportation ceased to function.

Slowly, a human tragedy was unfolding. Desperate migrant workers with their families began to trek home, to a land where certainty was more defined. Families began to trek across hundreds of kilometres without any state support. And all I could do was watch.

Three days earlier, I had completed a documentary on 'Riot victims and their children' on behalf of Delhi Commission for Protection of Child Rights. While shooting at Eidgah, many stories involved me emotionally and I began tentative dialogues with the inmates. There were calls coming in for support. I dropped at home to pick something and continue to my office. No sooner was I home that the head of the building resident welfare association appeared at my door with a meaningful smile. He said, 'So watch it,' he warned, 'all above sixty-five are the dangerous target!' My protests of 'but I'm only sixty-four' were lost on his retreating back.

So, despite what was happening in Eidgah to watching the thousands of hungry migrants on the road, I could do nothing except link NGOs to someone, who fell in the crack and couldn't access any other support; for I was the senior citizen in 'danger'!

When did this happen?

I could still run upstairs or charm exotic strangers. The voice exercises didn't ever let me down. Or the yogic stretches.

Maybe singles at tennis was a little too much; or cresting a ridge while chattering about the view.

But the lockdown was for all. Senior citizen or not. Twenty-one days of doing nothing, seemed insurmountably boring. But the fact was it was my time to catch up on so much more.

Books that were on my shelf and not yet read; the Brecht plays I had wanted to revisit for long; maybe read Shakespeare aloud. Exercise; have to go back to it. No chronological references to when last done, please. *The Habits of the Champion*, explained by successful astronauts (all those who have been there and back and are still sane) is the single rule. Fix a routine and follow it. Imagine following the tube of constricted passages within the spacecraft for days on end.

So, fix a routine. Easy on paper. But then there's reality. Juice, bacon and eggs, toast, marmalade and coffee at breakfast. Must go easy at lunch. Halfway into the bacon suddenly it dawned on me, how do we get to keep the supply lines going. Finally, coffee in hand the net trawler went at it. To organise the supply lines. All around there's trepidation. No one is sure. Not even Amazon; on whether they would be able to complete their orders. At least there was my wonder cook coming every day! Small mercies…

To be taken away swiftly! Again, by my nemesis, the building 'conscience'. The welfare association gentleman, with a maniacal smile hidden behind a mask—'No, we must not allow any domestic help, they come in from outside… after all we have to look after ourselves, above sixty-five…'

So, the domestic tasks one takes for granted now had to be done ourselves. Doing them seemed like an endless process. A new respect formed for those who looked after our homes.

The food schizophrenia continued…of not stopping to pick up bacon or burger patties, kebabs or…yet with a bleeding heart and ready voice waving the flag of dissonance for the migrant labour marching on roads or held up without any food. Still the government kept silent and the only directive was given to the state governments and civil society. While everyone floundered, it was only the civil society that kept providing food and other supplies to the miserable hordes. In a few days, the state government had its 'hunger centres' in schools and night shelters running and managed to reach out to many.

Yet what of my obvious double standards? Why couldn't I hunker down to just the basics that most of my migrant brothers would give a lot for! It reminded me of a time in Kolkata, when it was still Calcutta and we were in the university. We were helping a strike at a jute mill by doing a play. Everyone was very grateful and happy. After the play, I was getting ready to leave with my girlfriend, who had also performed in the play. Seeing us holding hands, a party official leaned in and advised, 'You are meeting the Dadas of the party; you don't want them to see you like this.'

In an instant, I let go of my girlfriend's hand but then I decided otherwise, laced my fingers through hers once more, turned our backs on the political agent and left.

With another extension of the lockdown, we are looking at a month gone past and everyone settled in their routines. How adaptable people are, they had realised that they had much to do in this lockdown. From getting to know each other to understanding our strengths and weaknesses to discovering hidden pools and resources that come to the fore. While nature seems celebratory due to this pause from human 'use'. The forests around where we stay are once more filled with birdsong. And the peacocks have returned!

Meanwhile, the central vista vanity project still continued, the government using its muscle to ensure no roadblock was more than just a sideshow—environmental, judiciary and all other bodies fell in line—while they shouted from the rooftops about how strapped they were for funds. New caring funds were being introduced with suspicious lack of public audit; and all I could do was to sit back and watch.

I guess this is the true import of Liberation.

> *'I and my bosom must debate awhile, and then I would no other company.'*
>
> —WILLIAM SHAKESPEARE, Richard III

The World We Lost

Reena I. Puri

Sixteen men sleeping on a railway track. Sixteen men tired, beaten, just wanting to get back home. The railway track was a safe place, the wooden sleeper, a hard but welcome bed and the steel track their pillow. All train services had been stopped, they knew. It was safe to rest and sleep, a numbing release from the pain of walking.

What they did not know was that freight trains were still running, carrying essential goods to different parts of the country. One came thundering down the tracks but not loud enough to wake them up.

The lockdown has thrown up many truths—some distressing, others encouraging. The sixteen men were walking to cope with the aftermath of the lockdown. The aftermath that took away their livelihoods, their dignity and made them orphans of the state, with the tag—migrants.

We are in a strange new world where everything that was normal has been turned on its head.

It is never going to be the same again.

The world, as we knew it, is lost. But, as I stand in my balcony and look up at the sky, it is the same. So are the trees, the flowers, the shrubs, the pair of wagtails hunting for worms and the cat washing its face, diligently. They all exist today just as they did yesterday or last month or last year. My vision scales the boundary wall and goes on to the broad six-lane road which just a month ago was thick with traffic. One could get the car out to go to work, exit the gate and then sit right outside the building for the next half an hour without budging. Today the road lies empty. All the vehicles that hooted and honked and snorted their way on it, are hunkered down in their stables. The riders, quiet in their homes. No excuses for road rage. The occasional ambulance whizzes by reminding me of the strange shadow that hovers over my species. Just my species. Is it our turn now?

We have silently watched as our companion species have slowly but surely been edged out of this planet. Some gone forever like the poor Dodo or closer to home, the magnificent Indian Cheetah. Forests destroyed, wetlands marauded, sea coasts plundered and the earth struck again and again to feed us and our vanities. Is there a rising? Quiet but determined? Can one hear the whisper of a virus? Who is the dangerous one? You or me?

A deep feeling of guilt holds me in its grip. I can see the thin face of a young girl in plaits, tears in her eyes, saying at an international forum, 'We are in the beginning of a mass extinction, and all you can talk about is money and fairy tales of eternal economic growth. How dare you!'

I work for children, have been writing stories for them for the last thirty years. Reliving myths, telling them of their glorious past, simplifying the great classics of literature, giving them the wisdom of our great men and women—have I done enough? Today, a child looks at me and says, 'How dare you!' And I struggle to respond.

It may be my imagination but the virus does whisper into my ears. Didn't you see this coming when they filled the waters with plastic and the flamingos stopped coming? Weren't you warned when the wildlife in your forests shrank in numbers as they were confined to tiny pockets of forests—beaten back when they dared to step out? You must have got an inkling when they mercilessly culled the dogs that you left on the streets and abused cattle that were sent out to graze on garbage. Didn't you see it when thousands of your own kind started walking home, in the searing heat of summer, to avoid starvation? No? You didn't? That is true blindness.

The lockdown, at the onset, did not bring home to me the full role of the virus. It is seeping in now and I feel very small. How I wish I had spoken earlier!

Fast & Furious

Snigdha Agrawal

Just about the time nature was going through a wardrobe change, casting off the browns and greys, replacing it with greens and reds, an invincible and invisible war was declared, on planet Earth. Like ants fleeing from their broken nest, people were seen running helter-skelter to malls and markets to stock up on essential items, following the announcement of the nationwide lockdown for twenty-one days. Never in our wildest dreams was this anticipated. First reaction was one of shock, fear writ large on faces, despair and stupefaction. No…this was totally unreal. Overnight everything changed, from 'living' to 'existing' in an unreal world.

Frustrations

For a sexagenarian/septuagenarian, not having lived through the world war traumas, experiencing this abnormal life-crippling phenomenon, seemed like being punched hard in the face. Holiday plans wiped out by the blackboard duster in one swift motion. Admittedly, the first disappointment in a series of many that were to follow. For travellers like us, planning in advance is but natural, to take advantage of cheaper rates offered by hotels, airlines or Airbnb accommodations. So as with applying for visas, paying up the steep non-refundable fees, an exercise all gone in vain, raising stress levels. Even then we stayed upbeat, hoping we would still be able to make it within the visa validity dates. That was not to happen, as Lockdown 2.0 and then Lockdown 3.0 followed, along a severity continuum.

Now looking back we realise it was a saving in disguise, as compared to the expenses that we would have accrued had we left before the lockdown, and like others, been stranded in foreign countries, cash strapped, anxious to touch home ground. Thus comforting ourselves, whatever happens, happens for the best! What if we had run out of medicines, evicted from hotels, left to fend for ourselves? Questions, for which there are no answers. Juxtaposition of thoughts surging in our minds. In retrospect, we felt lucky that our holiday plans had gone 'kaput'. The monstrosity of seeing bodies bagged and left on hospital floors, with no name tags, across the world, was a chiller. Then onwards, we started counting our blessings, thankful to be alive and kicking while seniors across the globe were falling like ninepins.

Fear

'Is *this* the Life We Really Want?' The answer is 'NO'. Living in fear, fear even to make eye contact with 'across-the-door' neighbours. Masked, gloved, opening the front door, one inch at a time, ensuring the floor elevator lobby area is deserted before placing wet and dry garbage bins for housekeeping staff to collect later would have looked ludicrous under normal conditions. But not then, crippled fear barriers clouded rational thinking, as if the virus would spread by exchanging pleasantries. A kind of maniacal fear afflicted everyone. And if perchance, timings coincided, doors slammed faster than lightning. Suspicion, another facet of fear dominated our minds. If there were no slamming of doors, again suspicion rose like acid reflux...must be under 'self-quarantine', with concurrent thoughts of its many ramifications. This despite the fact that many residents who had travelled overseas, just prior to the lockdown, were already in 'self-quarantine' mode in compliance with the advisories from the Apartment Association. But again, the 'what ifs' kept nagging...not entirely unreasonable, as we were seeing the end of the world not too far away based on the end of many.

Fatigue

Perhaps the biggest lesson learned from this experience was the need to be self-reliant. With the lockdown, and with all the services suspended indefinitely, we were totally flummoxed. At sixties, with health issues, how were we to cope with the household chores? But needs must when the Devil drives and so we drove ourselves to cook meals, clean the house, huffing and puffing, 'tired to the bone', dropping off into deep slumber at the end of each day.

After two weeks of popping paracetamols daily, to ward off aches and pains, sometimes even two, we gave up, and started online ordering for home delivery of meals from CureFit Kitchen, a health food restaurant. Some relief, followed by another huge one, this time exclusively for senior residents. Housekeeping staff, housed inside the complex—for maintenance and upkeep—were granted permission to help out in cleaning our homes. We took advantage of this, willing to pay whatever they demanded, obviously double/triple the applied daily rate. Once a week was enough for our home, with only the two of us, and zero outsider footfalls. The doorbell stayed in mute mode, except for delivery services. And to be truthful, this silence was getting to us, missing our family living just 5 kms away. Talking and seeing them on Skype was no compensation for the real human interaction. Exchanging notes on Sundays with family and extended family members living in the USA felt like reading a new chapter of the pandemic, a grimmer situation prevailing on their side of the fence. Festivals said, 'I'll pass!' Ram Navami, New Year, Easter, Ugadi, Rabindra Jayanti, birthdays, Mother's Day, just another day in 2020 Calendar. A Ghost World!

Freedom

With Lockdown 4.0 came a sense of hope. 'Freedom never felt so good' rang in our ears, with certain relaxations. And our first trip was to Toni & Guy, for a haircut after three long months. Every face 'Irwin Corey lookalike', anxious to transform to their former selves.

And overriding all this, now the bigger concern is for the millions of fellowmen, trekking, walking, riding on overloaded trucks, desperate to reach their homes, after losing their jobs. Not 'migrants' or 'refugees' as is being mentioned in the press. When did our own people moving from one state to another for better job opportunities earn this nomenclature? As I write, '*chapatis*' are being rolled out in every home, to feed the thousands of passengers, waiting at Whitefield Railway Station, to board trains bound for Andhra Pradesh, Orissa, West Bengal. 'No one has ever become poor by giving,' wrote Anne Frank and 'When we give cheerfully and accept gratefully, everyone is blessed', Maya Angelou. The need of the hour is to help the less fortunate, as we continue to stumble through this pandemic.

Weapons of Virus Destruction

Antara Dev Sen

'I think I have a headache,' said Tutu pensively. She narrowed her eyes and cleared her throat. 'No throat ache, though.' And then she coughed.

'Into your elbow!' I shouted, as I shot away from her. 'Let me get you a mask...'

'*Arre na re*... I was just checking,' she said with the air of a scientist pleased with her discovery. 'No throat pain.'

'Do you feel feverish?'

'Umm...maybe I should have a paracetamol.'

I felt her forehead. Warm. I felt mine. Warm. Too warm? My daughter Hiya rushed in excitedly: 'Do you have the Coronavirus TutuMa?'

'Of course she does not!' I snapped. 'Why don't you go finish your homework?'

'Because I have the *Korbo Na* virus!' laughed the ten-year-old. 'I will not!'

Life in the lockdown was getting testy. My dear childhood friend Tutu, who had come visiting for two days just before the country was locked, was also stuck with us in an endless wait in our little flat. With each passing day, her prayers—in diverse styles and several languages—were getting longer and more fervent, as were her phone calls to her family in Mumbai, primarily instructing them on household chores and hand-washing. Minati, our batty maid, periodically lamented that I had stopped her wanderings on the streets simply because I was jealous of her having *phoochka*s every day. Pratik, the man of the house, had taken to cooking exotic fare with a vengeance (and with every available dish in the kitchen). And our three cats seemed quite disconcerted by our constant buzzing around in what was clearly their home, routinely fixing us with the could-you-go-play-outside-please glare.

And after several weeks of being the bubbly indoor child who never steps out of the front door, Hiya rebelled. She packed her bags and declared that she was leaving.

'What?' we shrieked in unison.

'I'm moving out,' she said calmly, tucking shoes and toys into a big basket.

'You can't move out, you're ten years old!' screamed Tutu.

'There's a lockdown on,' said her father.

'*Ain?*' bellowed Mad Maid Minati. 'With so many shoes?'

'Where are you going?' I asked with manicured calm.

'Anywhere!' said Hiya. 'I have to go. I can't stand this anymore.'

And slinging a plastic rifle on her shoulder, with her backpack on her back, the basket spilling shoes and toys on her arm, she stepped out the front door pulling the big suitcase behind her. By the time we adults had gathered our wits and masks and slippers and had rushed downstairs, Hiya and her bags were at the gate of our housing complex.

'Stop! Child!' I shouted at the guards as I ran up like Maradona past his prime. They did. Hiya turned back with her bags, frowning furiously, and walked along the boundary wall. We pounced on her.

'Come let's go home, quick, before the Corona catches us.'

'Where's your mask? Don't touch anything!'

'What on earth were you thinking? You're ten years old!'

We crowded around her trying to take her bags, her hand, her unforeseen freedom, when she suddenly clambered up the bars of the fence and peered over it through the barbed wire onto the street. 'Uncle!' she called out.

Instantly, a couple of young uncles materialised on the other side of the wall. Ah, entertainment! Anything was better than lazing about in the capital's deserted streets in the afternoon of a heat wave.

'Could you catch my bag, please?' she said in respectful Hindi, as she readied to throw her backpack over the wall.

Quick as a flash TutuMa had climbed on to a mound nearby and was wagging a finger imperiously at the young uncles on the other side: '*Nehi pakrega! Bachcha panchil topkayega aur tumlog bag pakrega? Yaarki hai?* (You will not catch! Child will scale wall and you will catch bag? Is this a joke?)' Attacked by Tutu's fearsome Hindi, the uncle who was gearing up like Yuvraj Singh to catch the bag backed off. The other uncle spoke tentatively: 'There's a lockdown on *beta*, you can't be on the streets.'

'I don't care about the lockdown anymore—it never ends!' Hiya was ready to sling the bag at him.

'No, no,' yelled the terrified uncle, 'the cops will get you!'

'Absolutely,' I joined in. 'The cops will get you if you are out on the streets.'

A few other loiterers had gathered by then, all telling each other how miserable this lockdown was, and how it affects the minds of children. On our side of the border, an impressive crowd had gathered too, consisting mostly of guards and sweepers, all watching from a safe social distance.

'*Kya dekhta?*' Tutu thundered at them. '*Girao usko!* (What are you looking at? Make her fall!)' Of course bringing down a child from the top of a fence is not the same as bringing down a government—you don't try to 'make her fall'.

'*Utaro...*' I prompted.

'*Han han, utaro!*' the aunt commanded, '*sab log jao utaro.* (Yes yes, take it off. All of you go take it off.)'

The motley crew at home stood stupefied. The garrulous gathering outside continued to plead with Hiya, intermittently cursing the lockdown. Pratik and I tried to get her down, softly, lovingly, exasperatedly, furiously. Nothing worked. She stood on the summit, like Tenzing Norgay, holding aloft a backpack, in silent determination.

'*Chupchap dekhta?*' Tutu roared at the petrified guards. '*Chor dakat ayega aur tumlog etai korega, hain? Khara khara dekhega? Pakarke lao usko!* (Watching quietly? When thieves and robbers come you will do this, yes? Stand and watch? Go catch her and bring her here!)'

Admonished, one guard ventured towards Hiya. '*Ao Baby, nichey utro, ghar chalo...* (Come, child, come down, let's go home.)'

'*Arre, itna katha kyun bolta? Bachcha katha sunta? Upormey charo. Bachcha lao.* (Why talk so much? Does the child listen? Climb up. Get the child.')

At this, Hiya snapped out of her stubborn silence. 'No more Hindi, TutuMa!' she screamed. The impasse was broken.

We went home, bag and baggage, promising to let Hiya come down to our playground every day for some time. Maybe we had been too fearful. Too hasty. Too strict. Too unprepared. How long can you be in limbo? So okay, let her go get her fresh air. She would have to have her mask and sanitiser of course—the global weapons against COVID-19.

In India, a glorious ancient civilisation and a growing superpower, we were well-equipped to fight the Coronavirus. We had special weapons. The *thali*, for example. At the appointed hour, we the nation have crowded onto our balconies or terraces (or spilled out into the streets) to clang *thali*s as instructed. For extra power, we have blown conch shells, ding-donged bells, chanted mantras, sang songs. All potent moves to scare away the Coronavirus. *Arre bhai*, it has worked for centuries to scare away all kinds of terrifying troublemakers—from the wild boar to the gigantic elephant—of course it would work against a puny little virus!

Annoyingly, it didn't. So, we turned to the next weapon—darkness. We have a lot of darkness—all kinds of it, at home, in the villages, in our heads, our books, our ledgers, our policies, our minds, our conscience...in fact, if we wished to trade in darkness, we could perhaps be a world leader. So we brought out our weapon of mass destruction. At the appointed hour, as instructed, we switched off all lights. And lit a candle. Or a *diya*. Or many *diya*s. And fairy lights. And firecrackers. And a bonfire. We did some impressive tribal dancing around all that, bowing to the indomitable darkness.

The stupid Coronavirus was still unmoved. We sprayed our rooms with cow urine, and smeared ourselves with cow dung to purify our homes and strengthen our bodies, as instructed. This helped remarkably in physical distancing, thus keeping us safe. We chanted mantras, did yoga, drank gallons of warm water with lemon and most of the spices we had in the kitchen. We could practically feel the virus being killed right in our throats, or being flushed into our stomach where the little creep was hastily digested by our tropical tummies—experts at digesting all kinds of rubbish. We washed our hands. We closed down schools, colleges, offices, shops, the economy. Stay home, stay safe, we chirped.

And we did. Those of us who had homes. Home for many of us urban Indians was a small room shared between perhaps ten people, and a toilet shared between perhaps fifty. And for one in three Indians, home was a faraway village halfway across India. Locked out of work, these hungry, penniless thousands—men, women, children, the elderly—walked or cycled for miles across the country, being stopped and beaten up by the police on the way, dying of hunger, of thirst, of the heat, dying in road accidents as they plodded home or fell asleep on railway tracks. Dying of sheer exhaustion, dying of their motherland's intense neglect.

Which was the secret weapon that our great nation had? It made lakhs and crores of Indians vanish. So much easier to deal with a pandemic, when you have less people.

Anyway, I have to go. Time for my Corona puja. Women across Bengal, Bihar, Assam, Uttar Pradesh and Jharkhand are single-handedly warding off COVID-19 by their diligent worship of Ma Corona or Corona Mai. I need to do my share. You want to join in? Sure. Here, take this potato and stick matchsticks all around it…yes, it does look like a prickly ball. That's Ma Corona. Now put your hands together and sing with me...

See, we are well equipped to deal with COVID-19. Don't worry. Jai Hind!

Life in the Time of Corona

Mitra Phukan

These are surreal times. The rhetoric of war is everywhere. Fight the virus, honour the 'soldiers' who are at the forefront of the battle. A strange metaphor, for we all know that what we need are not warriors, but healers. Healthcare professionals who are working under great physical and mental stress, those people along with researchers on whom we pin our hopes. Still, the metaphor endures.

Nations are together in this, trying desperately to find a vaccine that will halt the virus in its tracks. Hope bubbles up in this murky mix, only to subside again. Nobody quite knows what's happening. The only thing that's certain is the number of infected, and dying. There seems to be no other news on this planet except the March of the Virus. In these dystopian times, every other activity, pursuits that celebrated human achievements, have been put on hold. There are no sports, we cannot go to halls to enjoy movies, music, theatre. Community activities are forbidden. The dead go on their way with very few mourners. The celebrations of Bihu are completely missing, and I worry about my musician friends who depended on the concerts of this season to see them through the rest of the year.

As we chafe inside our homes, as we wear the mandatory masks when we go out, we realise how aberrant this enforced lockdown—the strictest in the world—has been. We realise that truly, humans are social beings. Phone calls are not enough. I crave human company. I feel a great urge to rush into a crowded bazaar, jostling and buying things I don't need, throwing caution to the winds, just for the joy of social and physical proximity.

But, of course, technology has helped us through these days. Without it we would be truly lost. We can video call. Groups of friends meet on Zoom, and the laughter helps us through the loneliness of our lives. And yet there is fear and worry. A friend in New York, another in Mumbai, have fallen sick with the virus. We follow their progress with great anxiety.

Technology is helping us too, through the harshness of the situation. I am reading those downloaded books I never had time for, before. Those WhatsApp jokes bring a much needed smile into our lives. There are concerts where the participants sit and perform from different parts of the globe, joining their voices and instruments together to create the most beautiful music. For me this is a very moving thing. It is, for me, a metaphor of the human spirit, of the way in which people get together for a common good, the spirit which, in spite of everything, soars over all hurdles.

As lockdown after lockdown follow each other, there is now a great sense of restlessness, of wanting to get back to one's life PC. Pre Corona. In Assam, we are used to *bandhs* and curfews. But this is different. This is uncertain, sometimes life-threatening, and there's no knowing how long it will last. As supplies began to run low, I understood, just a bit, the insecurity that the hungry everywhere are experiencing. And though my larder was quickly replenished, I can't help thinking at each meal of those for whom even rice and salt is unavailable at this time.

It's been fifty-five days and counting since we've been locked down. I count myself among the lucky ones: I've been able to reach home just in time from a holiday outside the country. My family is safe, we are together in the same building. I sent off my help on paid leave, and cooked, swept, washed up and cleaned during the dusty days of the lockdown. No, I'm no superwoman. I did it all very shoddily and bad temperedly. Still, all of this has brought greater appreciation for the women to whom I outsource household chores.

As for work, it's been as usual. Most of what I do is online, anyway. In addition, I've been asked to give motivational talks to college and university students, for whom this is a time of great uncertainty. It makes me feel useful. I have been participating in online discussions about work—mine and others.

And there are economic worries. So many of my own have their own small businesses. They are hardworking, they have invested time, effort and their savings into their enterprises. They have been paying their employees. But they are not the ones who are posting pictures of the 'Planet Healing Itself'. They are worrying about how they will manage meeting their liabilities next month.

No longer do I look constantly at the graphs of the infected and the dead. I restrict myself to once a day. The terror of early days has given way to the grimness of the present. I can hear a couple in a neighbouring high-rise arguing at the tops of their voices. They have cabin fever, and who can blame them. But there's a sense of camaraderie too as people share apps that will fetch them fruits, and information about where in the neighbourhood veggies can be found.

The air is pure, nature sparkles. Yet the days pass in a haze of dull grey sameness. Just how many books, songs, movies can you consume, sitting at home, without company? I try to evaluate what I see on screens around me. Images of migrants going home, balancing bundles and babies, of being mown down by oncoming trains. News reports of people driven by hunger to break into houses and rob, sometimes injuring the people inside on the one hand. And on the other, on social media, images of people making chocolate cake, smiling into the camera as they cook really fancy dishes. No, I don't judge them. They are trying to stay sane too, and who knows which demons each person is battling at this time?

We're learning the art of minimalism. Cook with three ingredients, or even two. Filter coffee, my beverage of choice, has vanished from grocery stores, even online. I am making do, dismally, with instant. And yes, I feel guilty that I'm privileged enough in these times, to think of coffee.

Cleaning cupboards is a therapeutic activity, and I do it, even though they are now neat. But looking at the clothes, I wonder, why do I have so many? When will I ever wear them again? Some are new. Will the opportunity ever come to take off their labels and party in them? I shall give many away, along with a lot of utensils and crockery, to the needy when the floods, which are around the corner, come roaring in. I am paring down my possessions, my life.

I get nightmares. Nothing specific, just a nameless dread that stays with me when I wake up. I know others have it worse, they are battling depression. May they come out of it soon; may we all emerge sane and whole from this dark tunnel.

It is interesting to see how different people react in an unnatural situation like this. There are some who lock themselves into their cocoons, not really worried about others. And there are those who have taken it upon themselves to help out others, in however small a way, giving food packets, groceries to the needy and donating money. While I do not judge the former category, the work that these latter category of people are doing fills me with pride and hope for the future of humankind.

Janta Curfew

Debi Mukhopadhyay

Standing on my balcony
I feel the silence
Like a cosy blanket
(Not a shroud or pall)
And then the sounds
Come filtering in.
Birds chirping, flitting,
In great numbers
Towards the park
Where I usually walk.

All my neighbours
Are indoors
And what is more,
They are quiet.

The woman in Tower D
With a voice like a rasping knife
Where has she gone?
Is she savouring the silence too?

Today, for once,
The birds and squirrels
Must have claimed
The park as their own.
And in peace, I sit
And look at the blue sky,
Content to be.

The Eye of the Storm

Jael Silliman

I left Kolkata to visit my four-month-old grandson in New York—assured and grateful that my sister would spend a month of the two I planned to be away with our partially blind, ninety-year-old mother with whom I share a home. The Coronavirus was devastating Wuhan, a world away. At Kolkata airport, immigration officials were wearing masks; the crew were not. I put it down to some just being more cautious than others. I was unafraid and unshaken.

Soon after I arrived in New York, my friends were sent back from Italy to India and America. The grim dirge of news about how the Corona pandemic was ravaging Italy dominated global headlines. New York and India seemed far away from the crisis. Life here surged forward with no knowledge that the virus was stealthily making its rounds in and around the city. While I stayed mostly at home with my grandson, friends came and went—crisscrossing the city, the country and the world. The abnormally mild winter in New York ensured that people were out and about in restaurants, bars, museums and attended public events.

In a matter of days, the pandemic descended upon us with all its ferocity. Friends got sick, then colleges, businesses and schools were closed. Very soon the first few deaths became known—then the numbers grew exponentially and were represented in graphs. One New Yorker died every twelve minutes for three weeks from late March to mid-April. Living in Manhattan, not far from Mount Sinai Hospital, the unceasing, jarring sirens of the ambulances day and night, brought the magnitude of the crisis to my doorstep. Muscles tightened, lips trembled, afraid and shaken. I drew my grandson closer.

With alarming speed, we had become the epicentre of the pandemic. The lack of masks and preventive wear for health care workers, insufficient beds for COVID-19 patients, felt heinous. The city soon went into lockdown mode—people were asked to practise social distancing and to stay at home. Essential workers continued to make sure that groceries, chemist shops and more of a skeletal public transport system functioned. All of us are dependent on the essential workers so we can stay safe in our homes: they are the lifeblood of the city.

The ambulance sirens became incessant as hospitals around the city struggled to keep up with the Corona cases that are only beginning to abate. I read with trepidation and grief about the overflowing hospital morgues. I was shaken when a friend told me that several of her daughters' friends have been called for National Guard duty—their task was to collect bodies from homes, place them in refrigerated trucks to be transported to neighbouring areas for burial. The eerily deserted streets, the shuttered shops, the food lines and the number of people out of jobs was a harbinger of what is yet to come.

While trying to come to grips with the unravelling here, India's reaction to the pandemic unfolded. A day of curfew led to a complete lockdown on 24 March, with only four hours of notice given to the public. Flights and all modes of travel were cancelled making it impossible for me to return to Kolkata. I read the wrenching stories of hundreds and thousands of stranded migrant workers, with no jobs and food security, trekking hundreds of miles to their villages. Accounts of them being sprayed with disinfectants, facing police vitriol or dying on their harrowing journeys were profoundly unsettling. There were food lines several kilometres long in the cities—the wealthy were comfortably in their homes, some brashly displaying the elaborate meals they were preparing on social media.

I vacillated between enjoying the gift of more time with my grandson in New York and feeling anxious and a little guilty about my mother being on her own through this pandemic in Kolkata. Fortunately, my housekeeper, who works a day shift, agreed to stay in shelter with mum instead of being with her family. Each day I send her deep gratitude for ensuring my mother's well-being with grace and generosity. I snuggle in my grandson's soft tummy. He gurgles in delight. This unexpected, prolonged time with him has allowed us to develop a special bond.

I manically devour the news. I stray between headlines from New York and India. The grief around the mounting deaths in the city momentarily lifts at seven o'clock each evening by the wide outpouring of appreciation—applause, bells, honking and loud cheering honouring health workers, first responders and all those who keep NYC running. The situation in India feels murky. There is uncertainty about COVID and much that is unknown. The outpouring of support by ordinary people, religious institutions and the wealthy to address food insecurity does bring comfort. What is certain is that the economic and social repercussions of this pandemic on India will be devastating—perhaps even more than here in New York.

Questions to which there are no answers lash my mind. When may India relax its draconian lockdown of 1.3 billion people? How long will these uncertain times last? What happens next? When can my housekeeper go home to be with her family? When can I return home? When can people who are living in very confined spaces step out and resume their lives? What can I do to prepare for a more sustainable world ahead?

Through these dystopian months the daily walks in Central Park have grounded me—a reprieve I am privileged to enjoy. It is almost May—the white and pink apple boughs are heavy with flower, the whiff of Magnolia fragrance is in the air, tulips of many hues and bright daffodils in shades of yellow allow me to breathe deep and long with thanks on my lips and in my heart. As we take shelter in our homes, the world's air and water cleans and rejuvenates, the ozone layer slowly repairs and the animals and birds reclaim some of the land they were forced to abandon.

In my mother's lifetime we lived in more sustainable ways. We were embedded in local communities, depended on local markets and were more in harmony with the environment. There was less extinction of biodiversity and wildlife. Our relationships were more real than virtual. We could adopt the good values and practices of the past, harness technology for the public good, be mindful of all we consumed to reimagine the world we wanted to inhabit. What will my grandson's future hold? Our actions going forward will be his legacy.

Lockdown Musings

Deepak Hiranandani

1 May 2020

As lockdown 2.0 draws to a close, it is widely expected that in 'green zones' such as in my location, Panaji, Goa, the rules would be greatly relaxed for the next phase beginning on 4 May. I look back at this occurrence, the COVID-19 pandemic, as something most of us have never experienced before. A novel experience from a novel Coronavirus.

The world is the same, except that it isn't. We know now that all sorts of things which make up the quotidian fabric of our life can suddenly stop, or alter, considerably. A walk; shopping in the supermarket which happens to be in a mall (still shut and likely to remain so); hailing an auto or cab or taking a bus: these things are seen in a new light. Now, one is always conscious of the mask one is wearing and of the physical distance between other people in a queue or a shop counter or, well, anywhere...

The obvious set of issues which this lockdown has made us think about, among others, is the relationship between humans and the natural environment. Satellite images show that the air is clearer than it has been for many years. Following the Dhauladhar range being visible from Pathankot after decades, this morning we were informed that the peaks of Bandarpunch and Gangotri are visible from Saharanpur. The snow-covered Himalayas were seen from places hundreds of kilometres away in the plains—awesome. This is how India must have looked right through historical times until a few decades ago.

The non-human denizens of nature have become visible as they hadn't been for long. A rhinoceros strolling on a road in Nepal; penguins, blackbucks and ducks are among a wide range of fauna walking about the newly-deserted streets, roads and public squares all across the world (although there are reports claiming that some of these images are shown out of context and are misleading, some being older footage etc.). On a more sobering note, like this dreadful new disease, many diseases which have appeared in recent historical times have been linked with animals exploited by humans, whether captured from the wild or farmed for their flesh, milk or eggs. The Spanish flu of 1918, HIV, SARS, Swine flu, Ebola, Mad cow disease, MERS and now COVID-19 to name a few. From pathogens in wild animals consumed by humans to strains of pathogens from wild animals infecting farm animals, to mutations in farm animals with the mutant pathogen spreading like wildfire among thousands of animals crammed into sheds, their own immunity depressed due to the unnatural conditions and the high degree of stress: it's a sad story. And then there is the frightening looming spectre of antibiotic resistance in pathogens infecting humans, arising from antibiotics given to farm animals...

Our relationship with plants too, has come to the fore in unexpected ways. During the first few days of the lockdown, I always made it a point to have a wide variety of vegetables every day and to extoll the virtues of whole plant foods; I, was left scrambling under roadside trees for fallen green breadfruits and tiny unripe mangoes to cook: after all they were fresh edible plant foods, surely with some goodness in them. Lacking fruits except for one or two apples and pomegranates (no bananas—this for my daily banana eating self!) of which I had small portions each day, I picked up fallen '*safed jaam*', a semi-wild fruit which looks like waxy whitish *modak*s or garlic bulbs; while edible and not unpleasant they are not really delicious, tasting somewhat like a slightly sweet cucumber. But they played their part in my cherished variety of fresh vegetables and fruits every day.

Fortunately, I had plenty of dry supplies, but I shall never forget the poignancy of coming across three young men searching for a shop, any shop, to buy rice to cook. Not a single shop of any kind was open. I so wish I'd had the presence of mind to offer them some from my plentiful supply.

In addition to the seriously affected patients of COVID-19, some to the extent of fatality, we think of the lakhs of stranded migrant workers, of millions of lives disrupted, the colossal toll on economic activity, the tragic but mercifully relatively few suicides due to the disease or its disruptive effects—it seems now that the world will henceforth be thought of as Before COVID-19 and Post COVID-19.

21 April 2020

I hope the *koyal* finds a mate soon!

Since the last few days, every morning, e-a-r-l-y, a *koyal* (or perhaps they are different *koyal*s) starts cooing. Very, very loudly. It goes on and on, many a times, completely disrupting my sleep after listening to several minutes of the piercing siren-like sounds. Finally it stops: either the *koyal* tires itself out or has found a mate or gone to a distant tree to try its luck there. I'm assuming that the sound, extolled in our poetry and literature and lyric—indeed, I have used pictures of *koyal*s several times to illustrate videos of my Hindi-translated-Sindhi songs, which mention *koyal*s—is a mating call.

I gave up on my sleep for the first couple of days, which left me lacking in sleep and nodding off during the day to make up for it. Then I decided to hang around in bed and indeed sometimes I did doze off. But often, it was cruelly disrupted again because the *koyal* returned with its awful racket, which I suppose would have been awesome, a facet of living throbbing nature, if it had come at a time when one wasn't being disturbed.

It's not just here: a few days ago a friend from Kolkata sent a video of his beautiful leafy surroundings with a *koyal's* call. It was at six o'clock when he had heard it after a night of online work. I hadn't mentioned my *koyal(*s) to him yet but then, I did.

Today I'm grateful because I did get some sleep after being woken up; I even had a dream which I still remember. The *koyal* was back, of course, so I couldn't go back to sleep again as I had wanted to. But fortunately, it had come only just after my dream had ended...

Good luck to it, or them, in their amorous endeavours. *Pyar karo phoolo phalo lekin hamein sone do*.

28 March 2020

A day before yesterday, 26 March, on my fruitless search for vegetables in Panaji, within a radius of about 2 km, I found absolutely no open shop. On the deserted road, I came across three young men, who worked in a hotel or restaurant which was shut, had no food and were looking in vain for an open shop to buy rice. To my lasting regret only later did I realise that I could have given them rice and dal to cook but I wasn't able to find them again.

Later I came across a newspaper article online stating that Goa was reeling under the chief minister's 100 per cent lockdown stance, without milk, bread or medicines. Indeed.

26 March 2020

No vegetables available! Television shows that essential supplies are available in most places but here in Panaji the vegetable shops continue to be closed, seemingly in a 2 km radius of where I live.

Normally, I buy vegetables nearly every day during the course of my evening walk. Carrying three or four kilos, sometimes more, for over a kilometre must be adding to my fitness quotient. I eat many types of vegetables every day, small amounts of each. However, for the past few days I've been waiting till my stock is nearly finished before buying more, so as to minimise exposure to any novel Coronavirus there may be in the vegetable shops. Just when I was nearly out of vegetables the lockdown happened, and since then no vegetables or fruits had become available.

I still have a few potatoes, a couple of onions, a small and now precious tomato. The stem of an old cauliflower, withered as it is, could perhaps provide a few morsels.

Breadfruits lie about on the road, rotting. These had fallen before they could become ripe and usually people ignore them, while the ripe ones are sold, large and pale yellowish-green, having a delicately sweet flavour (but not really enjoyable as a fruit, they taste far better cooked) and a texture said to be reminiscent of *rawa* fish when the fruit is sliced and fried. I've never had that, but I find these unripe ones good to cook. When they fall in season, I often add a few chunks into my meal-in-a-pot dish. Well, now they'll have to play a lead role in the drama of my meal.

The cleaners on the roadside whom I asked said the vegetables come from neighbouring Karnataka and with the borders being sealed there is no supply. I tried at the official outlet of the Horticulture Department and yesterday, I even went to the shop at the state Krishi

Bhavan, but no luck. A passer-by and the cleaners said that all the shops are closed, so today, I didn't walk far and wide like yesterday.

I'll manage today, and tomorrow is another day. *Kabhi to sabziyon ka sooraj niklega*. Looking forward to *bhindi*s... bananas.

When Death Comes Knocking

Papia Roy

Coronavirus disease 2019, COVID-19 in short: such an innocuous, impersonal, harmless sounding name and yet, the very mention causes our hearts to race and panic sets in. More than 350,000 dead worldwide in a matter of months, and the numbers are steadily rising. It came upon us so suddenly that we never had the chance to give it an interesting name like Cholera, Typhoid, Ebola, Malaria, Pneumonia, Diphtheria *et al.* Perhaps later, perhaps someday.

It is raging through the US. Close to two million confirmed cases and more than one hundred thousand dead in three months, and that is definitely an undercount. There are more—many, many more. And there are going to be more—many, many more. Why? Because we do not want to be in a lockdown any more. Because we are desperate—every one of us, each for different reasons—desperate enough to throw caution to the winds. The US President and his party are thinking of the upcoming elections. The large corporations are desperate because they are losing money. Small business owners are close to bankruptcy. Farmers are ploughing over un-harvested crops. Dairy farmers are dumping milk, cattle farmers are culling their herd. Millions of unemployed people are facing homelessness and starvation. The lines at the food banks keep getting longer. And some are just desperate to flock to the beach and the park to enjoy the few warm months of the year. To go to the salon, browse the sales in stores, hang out with friends and family—cabin fever has set in and some of the psychologically fragile are crumbling under the strain.

The only voices of caution and dissent come from the frontline medical workers. They are screaming 'Stop, Stop' but no one is listening any more. The only people on their side are the old, the infirm, and society has silently written them off. The few voices of reason are already being drowned out in the clamour. A lucky few have the option to work from home but most of them know it is a temporary respite. They too are pushing back, their voices weakened by guilt.

By June 2020, we are all determined to open up, no matter what the consequences.

I sit in the relative safety of my house in Delaware and wonder how suddenly everything has changed. One moment we were blithely planning our future and now we are glad to be alive from one day to another. A few days ago, we were busy with work, family and friends. Now our solitary life is bumping around within these four walls. Our relatively normal existence has taken on a surreal quality complete with masks, gloves, sanitisers, social distancing, store pickups, food and grocery deliveries, hoarding and paranoia. As bad news keeps flooding in, the anxiety levels keep going up. An uncle is hospitalised in Mumbai at Hiranandani, a cousin is quarantined in her high-rise building, a friend's son (a doctor) is down with the virus, and another friend at an urgent care hospital is close to breaking point. We call everyone we know to check if they are okay. Our sons live far away from us and we are not sure when we will see them again. In our home country, the faces of migrant workers haunt our days and nights, a silent testimonial to a failed society.

Amid this chaos, a new challenge arises before us. We will need to move to Boston—a 360-mile drive through pandemic-ravaged states. A move from a sparsely-populated semi-rural area to one of the largest, most populous cities in this country. With about 700,000 people, Boston is struggling with more than 18,000 cases and 800+ dead. We will be in a totally unfamiliar new place where people are falling sick and dying at an alarming rate. We will be in an apartment full of young people, sharing elevators, escalators and walkways, commuting to the city by the crowded metro rail each day. The risk suddenly has gone up manifold, compounded by our age. Death is no longer an unexpected guest, though an unwelcome one.

What will my story look like by the time this account is published? Will I even be alive?

Young people think that the old make friends with death and gracefully exit this world. But in truth, one clings to life even more. Suddenly, the unknown expiry date begins to loom larger and larger. I think that is why the old don't sleep much. They are trying to extend every minute that is left to them. Your eyes dim, your hearing fails, your joints ache, lines on your metabolic report start to turn red, but you keep protesting—it is much too early—I am not ready.

Death is stalking our streets and we are doing our best not to catch his eyes. What then? Cower in worry and fear, sink into depression and despair, resort to drink and other pick-me-ups? I think not. Rabindranath Tagore says it best:

'I shall not fear, no—not I,
I shall not die daily deaths, before I die.'

Perhaps this is a reminder of how we ought to live. Not to take our lives for granted and squander our hours thoughtlessly, but to live each day as if it were our last. Time to dust off our keyboards, pull out our palettes and paintbrushes, put on our dancing shoes or anklets, and pursue all those dreams that fell by the roadside. Take the time to stand and stare and marvel at this beautiful world. Time to love, give and forgive. Time to find out who we truly are. Time to look back and redefine our path and our priorities. Tragedy and suffering can build or break us—our choice. We have no control over what life throws at us, but we can choose how to respond. Life is precious, life is a gift—make it count.

Solitary During the Lockdown

Nandini Dutta

We have never had to experience living with such an extended restriction on movement or social contact. As a child in Darjeeling, during the India-Pakistan War, I remember blackouts and curfew and how food was scarce. We learnt austerity and solidarity. This time around was not different and yet it seemed to me that the privileged and powerful had forgotten the marginalised and the less fortunate.

I am at a vulnerable age and have a complex medical history, which has made social distancing easy to practice and to follow. I have lived alone for the last sixteen years—loneliness has never bothered me.

As a teacher, I began to deliver classes online but it has always bothered me that while we can adopt new modes of teaching and adapt easily, what true education means eludes us. We do not inculcate values such as empathy or compassion, respect or tolerance. We impart information—and loads of it—but never practical wisdom. What if children learn to cook, do the laundry, learn the value of eating together as a family, stretch a Rupee and learn to live with less? What if we learnt to admire the gifts of nature? Would we be less educated?-

I have tried during the lockdown to renew my ties with my estranged daughter. There is a deep longingness, as I grow older, to share with her my thoughts, family anecdotes, songs, recipes. And to know that she is well and happy. And that we have put behind us the years of separation.

When a friend and colleague succumbed to the virus, I realised the frailty of life and the callousness of death. I admit that it overwhelmed me.

But I know it will end and life will begin again because it must.

Any Man's Death Diminishes Me

Navtej Sarna

This too shall pass, though the price will be high. Human nature will bounce back. Many sincere resolutions will be consigned to oblivion. We may even forget, once again, the bliss of blue skies and birdsong, or the beauty of a sunrise. We may again take good health for granted, our tomorrows as certain. Crowded supermarkets, mindless consumption, incessant shuttle flights and the pursuit of pelf and power may become our reality again. In the light of a new day, it is easy to forget the dark night: the twin tragedies of the Spanish flu and World War I gave way to the heady abandon of the Roaring Twenties.

But while we have the clarity that comes only when life hangs by a thread, let us reflect. It is clear that the world was unprepared for the COVID-19 crisis and we cannot be absolved of collective responsibility by calling it a Black Swan event—rare, near impossible and unforeseeable. As metaphors go, the Grey Rhino is more appropriate—the big obvious thing that was coming at us, and which we chose to ignore. The virus itself may be new, but our unpreparedness to deal with a global health crisis was staring us in the face. The warnings were clear: SARS, Zika, Ebola; each time we thought it was someone else's problem. The result is global chaos: stark shortages of hospital beds, ventilators, personal protective equipment; knee-jerk responses insufficiently informed by scientific guidance; disparate decisions on travel, trade, social distancing and lockdowns. Let's face it: somewhere along the way we lost the plot. Priorities got terribly distorted, globally: you only have to compare defence budgets with health allocations. Arrogance did the rest: countries forgot that nature could strike back, a pandemic could humble us.

Since this is no longer one country's problem, the response has to be both singular as well as collective. While health ministries will hopefully do the heavy lifting to correct distortions within, diplomacy too must play its role. Foreign policy is meant to better enable the alleviation of domestic concerns. This glib axiom needs to take real shape. For India—and we can take no comfort in the fact that other countries are worse hit—this crisis has put an urgent objective in focus: build a robust, affordable and accessible healthcare system. At present, the government health system is in a shambles and the vast majority of our 1.3 billion people cannot afford treatment at expensive private hospitals. International health cooperation can substantially bolster domestic effort in this regard. The foreign ministry can act as our sword arm to increase investment in the health sector, technology transfer and collaboration in manufacture of health equipment. It can also facilitate exchange of best practices in public and preventive health as well as targeted engagement with the

WHO, World Bank and platforms like G-20. Business as usual is no longer an option in the conduct of international relations: strategic great games, high-level visits, the arms race, trade wars and so on will sound hollow unless we also build in a response to this global tragedy. Diplomacy has to create conducive conditions in which money can be safely directed at people-centred sectors, in this case, health.

Too often, over the last few weeks, have I heard the cynical comment that more people die in India of TB than will die from COVID-19. That may or may not be true, but not a single person should die for want of care. To recall John Donne: '...any man's death diminishes me, because I am involved in mankind/ And therefore never send to know for whom the bell tolls; it tolls for thee.'

On Human Dignity

Navtej Sarna

'Grandpa buried his pa with his own hand, done it in dignity, an' shaped the grave nice with his own shovel. That was a time when a man had the right to be buried by his own son an' a son had the right to bury his own father.' So says Pa Joad in John Steinbeck's monumental protest novel, *The Grapes of Wrath,* as he digs a grave for his father even as the sharecropper family, like a thousand others, is on the road to California in search of work, driven off their land by the Dust Bowl, avaricious banks and mechanised agriculture.

In the end it is all about dignity: People reconcile to the inevitability, even the unpredictability, of death; but the details of departing trouble the mind. To die peacefully in one's bed surrounded by loved ones and not in the tortured blue-white light of the ICU is an understandable human desire. As is the yearning for a decent farewell, or burial in a pretty spot, or immersion in hallowed waters. It is all part of the final compromise with the unavoidable.

As in death so in life, men and women are at their most beautiful when they wear their dignity like a cloak that cannot be priced. When their values and convictions matter more than their bank balances. When they are remembered for what they did not for themselves, but for the needy stranger, the unfortunate other. When the hunger within them is for honest work and honest reward, for justice and fair play, for recognition of the humanity within.

Disease, like poverty, snatches at human dignity. Under the onslaught of COVID-19, hundreds are dying in the chilling anonymity of the isolation ward. Overcrowded burial homes are letting bodies decay in trucks in parking lots. Thousands are being given mass burials, each just a number on a television ticker. Fellow men are denying last rites to the dead for fear of infection. Children cannot attend funerals of parents; they watch them, like some surreal film, on Zoom.

We have also seen many journeys of sorrow. Like Steinbeck's sharecroppers, India's thousands, left without food, shelter or prospect 'streamed in on the highways and their hunger was in their eyes, and their need was in their eyes. They had no argument, no system, nothing but their numbers and their needs.' Human dignity cannot survive when a twelve-year-old girl, working in Telangana's chilli fields, dies trying to walk home to Chhattisgarh. Or a young man collapses on the Agra expressway, walking from Delhi to Madhya Pradesh. Or when several migrants, including a toddler, die in road accidents like dogs and jack rabbits on Route 66 in Steinbeck's novel. And still they walk on, bundles on their heads, babies in their arms, because even shorn of dignity they are human beings with 'a hunger in a stomach, multiplied a million times; a hunger in a single soul, hunger for joy and some security, multiplied a million times; muscles and mind aching to grow, to work, to create, multiplied a million times.'

Amid the misery, let us salute acts of dignity: doctors risking their lives despite being spat upon, policemen cremating persons whose next of kin could not reach, the doctor colleagues who prepare a grave for Dr Simon Hercules with their bare hands, after a mob prevents a proper burial. These men and women are like Rose of *The Grapes of Wrath*; having delivered a stillborn child, she saves a starving man by feeding him her breast milk. In that moment, she towers above human pettiness and greed. She becomes Mother Dignity herself.

Domestic Violence at the Time of the Pandemic

Lalita Panicker

The focus of the fight against COVID-19 has so far, correctly, been on preventive strategies, succour for the poor and migrant workers and the economic repercussions. But the pandemic has also thrown up several social issues, many of them gender-related. One of those, among many, is the issue of an increase in domestic violence, something that is kept hidden as far as possible in India even at the best of times. Women become more vulnerable to this at a time when they are literally trapped in their homes and kept away from people who could help them.

This violence has several dimensions. In the US, there are reports of abusers threatening to throw women out if they present any symptoms, genuine or not, of the virus. In India, such a situation can exacerbate the already weak position of women within the family—resources are normally limited for them given that they are usually economically disempowered and that their voices are not heard. In addition, given their marginalisation within the family structure, they are most likely to be forced to be caregivers for those who have contracted the virus and are quarantined at home. This makes them vulnerable to becoming infected and also to violence, if they refuse to carry out these duties.

Gender-based violence tends to increase in crisis situations like natural disasters, epidemics and conflict. There are reports that in February, China reported a tripling in domestic violence cases compared to the previous year on account of the lockdown then in place, according to activists.

For women in India, with the law and order machinery already overstretched, it is unlikely that domestic violence will be a focus at the moment. For those already in abusive situations, medical care and counselling will be difficult to find, let alone support systems even within the family.

The prolonged economic deprivation and fear of job losses often tend to create frustrations which fuel domestic violence. Kerala, now a model state in its handling of the virus, has had a history of domestic abuse brought on by unemployment and alcoholism despite its other enviable social indicators. So, the situation in less developed states—as people are driven indoors and facing economic disempowerment—can be imagined.

Parental homes, once a refuge for many battered women, are no longer an option as the elderly are most vulnerable to the disease and young people cannot take their presence or help for granted anymore. The victim of domestic violence now also faces the prospect of economic marginalisation as the labour market shrinks for women. So, in many ways, the woman is more dependent on her spouse or partner, even if in an abusive relationship.

In India, this is relatively uncharted territory but nevertheless one which merits attention even as the government grapples with other issues. It may come as a surprise to many, given its patchy track record on gender equality, that Uttar Pradesh has risen to the occasion and launched a special helpline for women victims of domestic abuse even as the state is floundering in other responses to the virus. The UP police has titled the initiative 'Suppress Corona, not your voice' as part of what it calls an enhanced response to cases of violence against women. This is online and accompanied by a picture of a woman wearing a mask. The underlying message is that wearing a mask to stop the spread of the virus should not mean that you cannot make your voice heard on domestic violence. The police has asked victims to call a helpline number and assured that women police officers will visit the victim in the event of a complaint. This is the sort of reassuring response that women victims need at this moment. It will not detract greatly from the other duties of the police and sends out the right message to abusers—that they cannot use the isolation and deprivation that women face as a result of the virus to use violence on them.

This sensitivity shown by the UP police to those who may need help but have fallen through the cracks in these trying times is commendable. It is something that other states could emulate and could bring about a modicum of hope and security to women facing domestic violence.

Fruits of Labour

Supriya Newar

Today I was determined to beat it; no no, not the lockdown blues and such. Just determined to beat all kinds of contestants that repeatedly got the better of me all of last week, each time I tried to lay my hands on the ripened mangoes.

You see ever since the lockdown began, I've moved from my high-rise living in South Calcutta to Salt Lake—a greener, semi-retired neighbourhood of the city—to be with my father. Structured and laid out in grids, each block in Salt Lake is quite *atmanirbhar* with its own markets, *mishti* and other shops, a community hall, ATM machines, its own set of stray dogs and its very own mango trees.

One such mango tree happens to stand at an arm's length from our house; from the kitchen window, to be precise. Not used to spending this much time in this kitchen (or my own for that matter), I had forgotten how full the tree looks when laden with mangoes, almost standing taller and prouder. In a world to which brakes have been applied, almost brutally, and an unknown, unrecognisable stillness has taken over the prevailing hustle-bustle, this mango tree gives out frequent assurances of life still being in order. It sways and gushes to the breeze, a *koyal* calls from it all day and the many mangoes hanging from it hold a sweet promise.

I watch the tree closely every day. Just like its neighbouring frangipani bush, which is full of buds that are waiting to blossom, the mango tree is making the most of the clear air and sunshine, its many fruits inching towards ripening.

But I'm not the only one eyeing the impending loot. Ever since the lockdown-life had started, more and more residents can be spotted at their respective terraces taking an evening walk or just enjoying the open expanse of a bluer-than-ever sky. And some of them have a pretty good view of the prized mango tree too.

By mid-May and the third phase of the lockdown, the mango tree is ready to yield and its many claimants are keeping a close watch. On day one, while chopping some vegetables we hear a soft thud and in less than a fraction of a second, spot a couple of greedy crows with their beaks firmly planted on the fallen fruit. By evening, I spot another ripe one, fallen on the ground, on which has descended an army of ants. My father looks at my crestfallen face and suggests if I want to have mangoes so much, why don't I buy a few from the fruit vendor? Wouldn't those be sweet enough?

I park that suggestion as a last resort, determined to taste at least a couple right from the tree. On day two, our cook and housekeeper, Aarti, and I, both are even more resolute. We hatch a plan that she'll keep an eye on any falling fruit while I'll make a dash for it. But as the lockdown is proving to us, man proposes and God disposes. Though she keeps one eye on the tree and sounds out an alarm right on time, '*didi...poreche...!* (Sister, it has fallen)' and I scamper down one flight of stairs as fast as I can, I'm beaten by a cycling milkman, who scoops up the fruit right before my eyes and rides away. To add insult to injury, Aarti lets out a full-throated laugh, as I sheepishly return empty-handed. Perhaps I should consider my father's suggestion and buy the damn fruit. Over the next two days, there are at least four more misses that I brave. I lose out to an on-duty policeman, more stray canines and a passing ice cream vendor. And very magnanimously, I hand over the one mango that I finally managed to lay my hands on to an elderly, portly neighbour to honour the *para* spirit. '*Ek i to bypar mashima...apni eta neyi nin...abar hobe to.* (It's the same thing aunty. You take this one. There will be another lot soon.)'

When the heat and humidity in the peak summer months of Calcutta becomes unbearable, a Norwester or a *Kalboisakhi* brings in much-needed relief. Dark ominous clouds gather, the breeze suddenly turns cool, winds blow at a reckless pace and the celestial drama that plays out in the sky ends in a short but fierce shower that shakes off the dust and humidity, at least for a couple of hours. It is one such *Kalboisakhi* that turns the tables for me too. No sooner had the winds turned wild, that a couple of the loosely hanging mangoes tear off from their branches and fall to the earth. With not a soul in sight, I march down triumphantly and collect them.

As I climb up the stairs, ready to beamingly show off my hard-earned booty, Aarti pales my delight. '*Ekhon khawa jaabe na. Fol ta shara raat jole thakbe—lockdown—er niyome. Shokale Shib thakur ke debo. Tar por shondhe bela apni prosad paaben!* (You can't eat them now. I'll soak them in water overnight as per lockdown rules. Tomorrow morning I'll offer them to Shiva and then you can have them as prasad by the evening.)'

My fruits of labour must wait.

Invictus

J. Alfred Prufrock

I hope 2020 remains the worst year of our lives. It would be terrible to face a time of greater fear and despondency.

The human race has been complacent. And hence unprepared. Sadly, even after The Virus stood forth in all its virulence, we, as a species, have not united in our efforts to survive. The one attitude that we seem to share is escapism. 'It can't happen to me. Even if it does, it won't be critical. Even if it gets a little tough, I'd pull through.' And death laughs a great silent laugh that swallows the light.

I love my family. And I fear for them. Which is why I have erred on the side of caution. Much better to stay at home and go without, than to step outside and vanish like a puff of smoke.

It seems sadly appropriate that Basu Chatterjee passed away during the lockdown. His gently paced romances set in middle-class Bombay (long before Mumbai) evoked a gentler pace, a kinder space, when time was a promise and not a threat. And much of the shooting was done outdoors, on wide roads, on open beaches, on Marine Drive and in little corners of the city. They all seem so spacious now, uncrowded, unhurried when we see them through the lens of the forty-odd years that have passed.

Television played those scenes over and over again. Amol Palekar walking down Bandra lanes lined with bougainvillea, or with Tina Munim on a beach. In *Manzil,* the picturisation of Lata Mangeshkar's version of *Rim jhim gire saawan* is one of the most beautiful depictions of Bombay in the monsoons. We see the majesty of the sea against the stone breakwaters, we feel the magic of the raindrops on our faces, we can almost smell the petrichor as the first sheets of rain wash the roads clean. It celebrates the open spaces and the openness of the city.

And we sat inside our homes, behind our locked doors, and yearned for that freedom again.

Our hardships, of course, were not real. They were mere inconveniences. Tragedy played out outside our doors. For the first week or two, our hearts shrank at the thought of those who fought the disease, fought death and the many who lost. We read about a world unsure of how to treat the disease, or how to stop its spread. We read about old people dying alone because their loved ones could not be allowed to see them. But the worst was yet to come—we read about thousands of poor workers and their families walking hundreds of miles to reach home. We saw children stoic in the face of heat and hunger, the cracked and bleeding feet, the wordless suffering. It got worse. Even when trains were arranged to take them home, there were stories of long hours on lost tracks, without food, without even water. I know for a fact that my young colleagues in the districts stepped in to help and feed these trainloads, and to send them home safe. But still the news came, of deaths from hunger, thirst and sheer exhaustion. The sadness stayed within us like a dull ache, a foreboding, sorrowing at our futility. We gave money to salve our collective conscience, to soothe our grief. We gave of our time, our effort. We tried to stop the hurt.

And still it got worse.

Even as nature brought mankind to its knees with a microscopic virus, it unleashed an awe-inspiring, terrifying dance of destruction with Cyclone Amphun. In Odisha, which suffers from this fury every other year. And in Bengal, where the most terrible cyclone in nearly 300 years razed the southern half of the state. The economic tragedy of the lockdown became even darker. The Sundarbans were devastated. Fields were flooded with salt water. Homes were destroyed. Electricity, roads, drinking water were disrupted. People across seven districts in the path of the storm lost homes and livelihoods. In Kolkata itself, old people lived without water or power until trees could be moved and wiring restored. The cyclone felled more than fifteen thousand trees across the city alone, trees that smashed walls and tore up roads as they fell. And my city's green and shady spaces died along with them.

Bengal rallied after the cyclone. Even as debates raged in the media over the quantum of damage and the amount of aid required, common people joined the administration in helping. They took food, clothes, medicines, tarpaulins to the villages. Life staggered back towards normal. Towards the new normal. Offices started up. Planes flew again. Shops and markets reopened. In the midst of all this, we had to cope with the death of a dearly loved member of the immediate family.

So could the shades of sadness fade at all? For a while, it felt like they did not.

And yet, perhaps they did.

Did the virus, and the lockdown it brought, strip away the parts of our lives that were unnecessary? As one meme put it, it was strange that the world economy was shattered because people started doing without what they did not need. Oversimplification? Maybe, maybe not. We couldn't go out in the evenings, we could not party with friends. We stayed home, we read books, we watched movies. People tried to sing, they learned to play musical instruments. Many sketched, painted. Some knitted, crocheted. We spent time with our families. Yet, for fear of infecting my parents, I have visited them only once since lockdown started, though I have spoken to them every day, and seen them up close on video calls.

We learned to talk again. Talk to our families, to the loved ones we live with. And we learned to value talking to friends, whether on the telephone or over video calls. The world grew smaller.

The world grew greener, too. We rejoiced as the air grew cleaner, even as we laughed at the satirical claims of Kanchenjunga being sighted from Kalyani. We wanted to believe that the animals were coming closer to us, even though we knew that they were just more visible in deserted towns and fields.

We found peace in quieter days and nights. We found silence in the darkness, a silence that had long been lost to traffic and to machines. We found birdsong in the quiet mornings, as the *koyal* that had started calling in late February sang its heart out all through May. Music would always play around me, but now, as I walked in endless circles around our building, I started really listening to music again. Remembering 'lonely men in shirt-sleeves/ leaning out of windows', I too found peace by an open window, as cool soft breezes from unseasonal showers lifted the curtains.

I learned to savour solitude.
And peace came dropping slow.

Rabindranath summed it up (as he summed up so much of our existence) when he wrote, *'Achhey dukkho, achhey mrityu, biroho dohono laagey / Tobu-o shaanti, tobu aananda, tobu ananta jaage'*: Grief exists, and death awaits. Parting scars the heart / Yet amidst this, peace exists and joy arises, within the infinite.

Always Half Full

Mousumi Sengupta

I have always been God's favourite child. Either my dreams come true or I have this ability to relish and cherish all the experiences that I go through, including the 'not so good ones' too! It is really a win-win situation for me. Therefore, at the very onset, I would like to mention that I will concentrate fully on the positive side of this lockdown period.

When #COVID-19 struck the planet, I was understandably heartbroken! A 'never witnessed before' pandemic was engulfing the world, about to affect millions adversely. But I soon realised that every cloud has a silver lining. To arrest the acceleration of the deadly virus from affecting us, the never-ending lockdown was announced, albeit in instalments, and this delighted me to no end! This, of course, falls under category 1 of one of my dreams coming true!

My family, my dearest ones, my favourite people could now spend time with me 24×7, God knows for how long! Being an eternal optimist, I decided to focus on all the positives associated with this lockdown, and simultaneously I continued doing my bit for society—the aged, the needy and those in great distress.

My husband and daughter were always by my side physically. After years, we had all the time in the world for laughing together, talking, eating, having fun together, for great lengths of time. Sometimes even cooking together, discovering new facets of each other and oneself, planning the future without realising what exactly this pandemic would do to us. So even though COVID-19 destroyed the vacation we had planned in three countries, it failed to dampen our spirits.

We picked up some new concepts during this period. Online seminars (webinars), online live entertainment and most importantly online classes for my little one! Faces of forty children squeezed into the small screen of a tablet, interacting with their teacher on several subjects! While my daughter is not very fond of attending school, this novel concept somehow attracted her! There she was, bang on time, in front of the smart screen!

We tried out new, innovative recipes practically every evening. We got to taste *phuchka*s prepared by my sixteen-year-old, definitely a delicacy and a rare commodity in COVID-19 times, an exotic biryani and some delicious burgers for breakfast, thanks to hubby dear! While on the one hand we were experimenting with new recipes, on the other we continued to try and help those suffering miserably.

From the very beginning we kept receiving numerous calls from all over the world from panic-stricken friends and even from unknown people. The elderly parents of some were based in Kolkata and they were in great distress. Some were octogenarians, unable to procure food or emergency medicines during the lockdown, some critically ill were refused admission to hospitals owing to lack of beds, and others were absolutely disheartened, demoralised and in great fear! There were other cases of getting permission for travelling from one city to another, owing to a dear one's serious illness or even death!

We, as a team, decided to be with these people. My husband being a senior bureaucrat had to focus largely on his 'job'. Being reasonably resourceful, we managed to ease the pain of nearly all those who approached us. This was really a golden opportunity to support those in distress. In the bargain, we benefitted by gaining deep satisfaction, love and blessings! It was also very flattering to hear your own eulogy from a stranger in another country, who has not even met you! At some level we were happy that we might be earning 'good karma'!

I must mention one specific incident that had given us tremendous satisfaction and, much more importantly, saved lives.

We got to know unofficially that a train was travelling from Bangalore to South Bengal with migrants. My domestic help's sister, Durga, was one of the passengers along with her eight-year-old son. The passengers were neither allowed to carry food nor were provided with water! Inevitably, within twenty-four hours, there was utter confusion and chaos amongst the passengers. The panic-stricken travellers went wild; they started squabbling among themselves. They were exhausted, hungry and understandably fuming! The ravenous children were falling ill. They could be heard howling for food. They would soon collapse! The inhuman treatment faced by them was unbearable, to say the least. They were not even allowed to disembark, so the question of procuring food did not arise! To make matters worse, once the train entered West Bengal, it was diverted to North Bengal, which was completely in the opposite direction from their scheduled destination!

We were being constantly updated on the phone by Durga. We could not tolerate this any further. Atri, my husband, swung into action, contacted the district administration, briefed the officers about the plight of these miserable ones and requested them to come to their aid. Soon the district officers responded magnificently. The train was stopped midway, some food (buns, chips and fruits) for thousands was arranged in record time, the passengers were offloaded. Buses were arranged to take them to their homes in South Bengal.

Apparently the food provided came as a boon for the travellers, as if it had created magic, especially amongst the kids! They gorged hungrily on the unexpected bounty. It was so heartening to picture the smiling kids, fully satisfied after some food at last. For me, this incident was definitely a highlight of the lockdown period. Durga now wants to visit us in Kolkata to express her gratitude, in the form of a large, fresh Hilsa!

COVID-19 attacked the human race without discrimination! Daily updates about the number of deaths across the globe, the deaths of people known to us, the unexpected deaths of youth, the worldwide chaos regarding shortage of beds in hospitals, the unattended ailing, the relatives of COVID-19 victims who could not even catch the last glimpse of their loved ones before their cremation, the brave doctors and nurses contracting the virus, the utter ignorance of the people...such news made us extremely depressed but we were helpless!

However, the most significant incident of this period was yet to come! The incident that left me traumatised, helpless and vulnerable. The incident that left my heart bleeding! It was waiting at the threshold and quietly crept in!

My ailing mother was hospitalised at the very beginning of this lockdown period. Our daily duty was to visit her, braving all odds associated with the lockdown. In addition, there was the fear of getting infected during our visits to the hospital. On seeing us, invariably her face brightened up! Her smiling face made us forget about all our worries. This was so rewarding, so comforting! She returned home soon, but had to be rushed back to the hospital within a day or two.

In the midst of all this, West Bengal was hit by *Amphan*, the most destructive cyclone in 300 years! It hit our state at an unthinkable velocity of 150km/hour! It shattered and destroyed so many lives of both human beings and animals, properties, natural resources, plants and trees! Rural areas of South Bengal were completely wiped out (15,000 trees fell in Calcutta alone!). We personally experienced horror! The sway of our high-rise, the lash of the wild storm on our glass windowpanes, the non-stop roar of the wind and the unexpected flood right inside our living room and kitchen! The electricity and internet connections were down for days on end! *Amphan,* of course, destroyed our morale too. While we were struggling with COVID-19, *Amphan* gave us our last blow! Our struggle trebled, but life has to go on.

After more than a month of battling an infection, my mother was well on the path to recovery. So while the lockdown was about to end on 1 June, we were preparing to bring her back home. But Lady Luck refused to smile on us. On 31 May, my beloved mother left us forever, after putting up a tough fight for forty-three days! Yes, I lost her during the lockdown!

I had confessed earlier that I am an eternal optimist. Trust me, this incident too, left me happy! Look at the positives...thousands across the world are dying an early death every day, thanks to COVID-19. Most of them are much younger than my 80-year-old mom! My mother had a wonderful, fulfilling life; she was relieved of all her pain and finally she joined her loving husband to be pampered in heaven! Oh yes, deep down it made me so happy!

So that's my lockdown story. Good and bad, ups and downs, gain and loss, life and death. We are part of world history now; we are witnesses to a watershed in world history! Is the lockdown over? Not sure. Will it be back in its full-fledged form? No idea! But if you ask me, this lockdown in my experience has been eventful, constructive, fulfilling, satisfying, filled with rich experiences— both sad and happy. So for me the glass is always half full...it's three cheers for the lockdown!

The Accursed Wednesdays of COVID-19 Lockdown

Debanjan Chakrabarti

Wednesdays are cruel. They always have been. Since the onset of the COVID-19 pandemic, when home is all that remains of the world, that day bang in the middle of the work week appears more ominous. It inevitably is the longest day of the seven when anything that couldn't possibly go wrong also goes wrong. Wednesday, 27 May, was no different, keeping up the trend of the other dozen or so preceding Wednesdays since the lockdown began in late March. Work calls and online meetings had dragged on till well past 8 pm when I noticed a series of missed calls from an unknown number and one from *Chhotomashi*, my mother's youngest sister, on my mobile. This venerable aunt of mine is known for not wasting time on niceties and would never call, unless it was important. I also hadn't noticed earlier that another ominous storm was busy balling up its fists on the southern horizon.

I rang up the unknown number first. My mother picked up the phone. Over a poor connection and the chatter of a lot of voices in the background, I detected clear panic in her voice. Their building—one of the oldest multi-storey apartment buildings of Kolkata, at Ballygunge Phari—had caught fire. All fifty-five apartments had been evacuated and several fire tenders had arrived. There was of course no electricity and…the crotchety network snapped. I tried again. The call wouldn't go through. The reason for this poor connectivity was buried in debris left behind by the happenings of the previous Wednesday.

* * *

20 May was the ugliest Wednesday of the century for south Bengal. *Amphan*, a category-four severe cyclone, rampaged through Kolkata like an angry and spiteful sea monster from the dark depths of legends.

It was like nothing I've experienced before. I am a bit of an adrenaline junkie. I like extreme roller coasters. And bumpy flights. But *Amphan* scared me like nothing I have known in my not-so-inconsiderable years on this earth.

Terrifying and spectacular, it was nature's theatre at its most capricious. The storm tore through the city at well over 130 kmph. I have driven at that speed but had no idea what relentless gusts feel like for over four hours. The angry wind clawed and banged at the windows of our third-floor apartment like a poltergeist, threatening to rip them apart. The mighty rattle of the windows and doors was all but drowned by the feral snarl of the storm. And that sound was not just what you sensed at the ground level, or even at three floors up. The horror of that ungodly sound lay in its dimension and depth.

At the treetop level, there was the obvious shrill noise of wind and rain—coming in from the north-east and almost parallel to the ground—whistling through the clumps of trees, their foliage and the gaps between buildings and lampposts and railings, whooshing across the open waterbody that lay ahead, whipping up waves that were entirely disproportionate to the size of the pond. But that was a sound I am familiar with, from countless Nor'westers, or *Kalboishakhi*s, the poetic sounding Bengali name that aptly sums up the fearsome nature of those short but intense summer evening storms.

What was unusual this time was the deep-throated growl that came from above. It was like the whine and screech and thump of a million helicopter gunships hovering above. Think of the Ride of Valkyries scene from *Apocalypse Now* and scale it up a thousand times. It was ominous and sinister, an enraged reprimand to humankind for the countless sins of polluting the air, water and earth, a savage reckoning for the wanton destruction of creation.

The morning after revealed that much of the civic infrastructure in Kolkata and neighbouring districts of North and South 24 Paraganas was smashed—over 5,000 large trees were uprooted in the city alone, the Sunderbans lay ravaged beyond recognition and Bengal's heart was pulped and mangled. Large swathes of the population were to go without power, regular water supply and mobile connectivity for the next fortnight and more.

* * *

I gave up trying the unknown number and called my aunt. She summed up the situation for me. At around 7 p.m. a fire caused by an electrical short circuit had broken out in my parents' apartment building. The acrid smell of burning plastics and rubber and a neighbour frantically banging on their door had alerted my parents to the fire. Because their flat was upwind, they hadn't quite realised how bad the situation was. My father is a COPD patient with a pace-maker and has a neurological condition that has started to afflict his balance and gait. As soon as they stepped outside, they were engulfed in thick fumes and saw flames licking at their doorstep which would have proved disastrous for him in particular but for a brave young neighbour. He had picked my father up and carried him in his arms seven floors down. My mom's mobile phone had run out of charge.

I decided to rush to Ballygunge Phari. The streets were deserted and the scars of *Amphan* were everywhere. And another feisty Norwester was brewing: I could see massive columns of dark clouds with cobwebs of lightning flickering on the marching formations as I raced down Gariahat flyover. I arrived just after the fire had been put out. It took us over thirty minutes to climb up seven storeys with my father. We got inside the flat engulfed in pitch darkness. The floor was flooded with the water used by the firemen to douse the flames. And we could feel debris floating on the ankle-deep water sloshing around.

My mother and I start mopping the water. After an hour and half of back-breaking work, we are not wading in water anymore. My plan was to bring my parents back to our place for the night, but both of them were in a state of shock and insisted on spending the night in their own apartment. I gave up arguing with them and helped them settle in for the night. I then visited some of the neighbours, most of them elderly and frail and good friends of my parents. In their deep empathy I saw the reason why my parents felt safe and cocooned in the bosom of this community even in their hour of deep distress. Tomorrow will be another day, I said to myself as I started making my way back home to Prince Anwar Shah Road.

And then the storm hit me. The Nor'wester that I had ignored on the way in was far from over. South Calcutta was wrapped in darkness. Giant arcs of lightning still streaked across the lowering sky every few seconds, the boom of thunder following a few seconds later. The rain pummelled the windscreen. Many trees that had just about survived *Amphan* were heaving perilously like inebriated giants all around me. Two of them crashed, missing my car not by much. It felt as if I was on the set of a Hollywood disaster movie. Or was caught in the vortex of an ending Shakespearean tragedy that kept peeling layer after layer of human despair. And as if on cue, the wind howled hauntingly like a Greek chorus.

Pandemic Protection

Mangala Gouri Chakraborty

I come from a line of TamBrams
Who have rules for every event.
So for visits of condolence,
My grandmother, a matriarch,
Inculcated in me these rules:
Don't touch, don't sit, don't talk—she said,
Leave your slippers and wash your feet
Before you come inside;
Wash hair and bathe and scrub your clothes
And then relax at home.

So after I came home today
From the bank I went to for cash,
I knew just what I had to do.
I hadn't talked or sat or touched
(Excepting the ATM cash)
Returning, I followed the rules,
Left my slippers and washed my feet
Before I came inside;

Washed hair and bathed and scrubbed my clothes
And then I sat, relaxed.

This moment in time is, I feel
A phase of communal mourning.
We all must grieve the loss of life
As we knew it, some time ago.
Public places have to be shunned;
Meeting friends at road side cafés;
Visiting, travelling, shopping:
All that filled each day of our lives,
We have to give up—to survive.
Is life then, worth this sacrifice?

The Dispossessed

Mangala Gouri Chakraborty

They left their homes
They left their wives
Some women left
Their peaceful lives.
Carved out a niche
Working for rich
Entitled folks.

Happy to send
Back cash to fend
Off hunger pangs.
They provided
Hard cash instead
Of fathers' touch
Or mothers' care.

COVID- 19
Now changed the scene.
They lost their jobs
They lost the cash

They lost the place
They used to stay:
Were shooed away.

And now in hordes
They crowd the roads
Walking all day
Making their way
To loving homes
Bearing as gifts
The virus.

A Divine Dilemma

Amit Dasgupta

I heard about it from someone, who insisted he was in the know of things because he had some kind of direct line with The Powers That Be. He said so in hushed whisper, eyes closed reverentially and index finger pointing upwards. The gesture was prone to interpretation but Manik Biswas was known to be God-fearing and wished no one any harm. When he was not at his liquor store on Ballygunge, he would spend his time in prayer and chanting, with his wife beside him and their two toddlers on their laps. His chanting was an assault on the eardrums because he was as tuneless as I am but that's another story.

I have known Manik for around four decades and have never seen him consume alcohol or imagine things, consequently, in drunken stupor and so, I was quite intrigued by what he had said. All of this was done over the phone and some via email because the lockdown prevented us from meeting.

He told me he had got to know that the Triumvirate had convened an 'extraordinary general body meeting', where the presence of all members was mandatory. The meeting was presided over by Brahma and co-chaired by Vishnu and Shiva. Kartik was appointed as the Secretary and tasked with taking notes and preparing the 'minutes of the meeting'.

At the appointed hour, the meeting commenced. Clearing his throat, Vishnu expressed satisfaction that there were no abstentions and with a grim face, he announced that there was a single agenda item: What would happen to Durga Puja this year? A gasp followed, which was understandable because to even ask such a question was blasphemy. This was a tradition that predated time itself.

The loud murmurs grew quiet, as Ganesh turned his impressive head and said, 'Order! Order!' Vishnu continued with a thank you nod and said, 'The lockdown and social distancing has triggered a dilemma of extraordinary proportion and of a kind we have never witnessed before! I ask you to ponder, when would the *pratima*s be ready? Who would make them? What about the puja *pandal*s? Who would construct them? What about the puja markets? Who would open them? What about the crowds and the *dhakais*? Who would permit them? What about the *mishti* and the *ranna bati*, the *bhog* and the cultural programmes?' He stared glumly at his audience and whispered, 'We have a disaster!'

Manik told me that there was deathly silence all around, as the members allowed the import of what was said to sink in. Only Mahishasur seemed elated. He twirled his moustache and ran his fingers through his freshly-oiled hair and said, 'Finally! A year when Durga would not beat me to pulp! It has been embarrassing and insulting! I am fed up with these stage-managed WWF-style fights! A celebration is called for, I'd say! Long live the virus!'

Saraswati, known for her wise counsel, and Lakshmi, the Treasurer, dismissed Mahishasur's statement with a contemptuous wave of their long fingers and manicured hands. 'No time for jokes,' they said, 'what about a virtual puja and an online celebration? New times, new approach, cost-effective as well.'

The buzz and the murmurings started again and though they were getting louder by the second, Ganesh did not intervene to silence them. He knew that this was indeed a complex issue that required out-of-the-box thinking. Tradition was tradition and unless it was protected, nurtured and kept alive, people would lose their identity. They would forget who they really were. Ask any Bengali and they would tell you, without Durga Puja, we are nothing. And it is the same for the other twelve festivals we celebrate through the year. Thirteen festivals in twelve months define us! As simple as that. But it was Durga Puja that stood out as the mother of all festivals.

Birendra, who was a special invitee to the meeting, stood up and said, 'I have been recorded and am available on YouTube. Mahalaya can go off without a glitch.' There was a general murmur of assent. Birendra resumed his seat and adjusted his starched *dhoti*.

I was truly impressed by the kind of detail Manik was privy to.

'Do I take it that we have a consensus then?' Vishnu enquired from the congregation, 'We modernise, we embrace technology to keep tradition alive!'

As the lead participant in the festival, Durga felt obliged to comment. 'Virtual and online are not the same thing,' she said, with a sulk. 'I mean if I have to beat up Mahishasur, it is so much more *alive*, if I am able to do it in multiple places at the same time!' Mahishasur stared at her coldly, exposing his biceps and triceps.

Shiva decided to interject as co-Chair. He always liked to have the last word and ensured that Kartik dutifully recorded his interjections accurately. 'I think Durga is right. Online is only second best to the real thing. But desperate times call for desperate measures. As Vishnu has advised, we need to think afresh and anew. We have a great and unique opportunity to do so. Let us portray Mahishasur as the Coronavirus and Durga as the antidote that we have all created.'

Manik told me there was stunned silence followed by resounding applause at this extraordinary suggestion. A veritable game-changer, some called it. The meeting ended with a vote of thanks that Ganesh delivered with much aplomb.

I stared blankly at the phone, wondering what Manik would say next. 'When the lockdown and social distancing are eased, we need to catch up over a drink,' he said, before disconnecting.

Pen Pallery in the Time of Corona

Bunny Suraiya

I must have been around fourteen or fifteen years old when I made my first pen friend. I was taking French classes at the Alliance Française in Calcutta and felt it would be cool to have a French pen friend on whom I could practise exciting phrases like, '*La plume de ma tante est dans le jardin.*' (The pen of my aunt is in the garden).

I don't remember how one found pen friends in the era before the Internet, but somehow I did find a nice-looking French boy named Gayan. An unusual name, I thought, vaguely expecting almost every French boy to be named Francois or Pierre—or at the utmost, Guillaume.

But Gayan? What was this? Some Indian boy masquerading as a French *garçon,* even though the photo accompanying his first letter showed a suitably blond lad? It turned out that Gayan's parents were Indophiles and had named their son after the Sanskrit word for 'song'.

Just my luck. I wanted to know all about Napoleon, whom I admired madly, and the fashions of Coco Chanel and the history of the Eiffel Tower and what it felt like to promenade on the fabled Champs Élysées—while my pen friend wanted to know all about Indian gods, goddesses, festivals, rituals and boringly on and on! It took about three exchanges of letters for our pen friendship to fizzle out—I suspect to our mutual relief.

Fast forward to 2020. Jug and I have by now become intrepid and frequent travellers, who fell in love with Italy about a dozen years ago and who look forward to our holidays there every summer and autumn—and sometimes spring.

I love the country and culture so much that last year I started taking twice-weekly Italian lessons from an Italian teacher named Alessandro, in order to make our travels more enjoyable. Following our tradition, last November we booked our summer holiday in Italy, planning to arrive in Roma, then move on to Bologna, Milano and Bergamo, from where we would take our flight out of the country.

And then Corona struck. Italy got very badly hit and shortly after, all international flights got cancelled.

With a heavy heart I wrote to all our B&B hosts, in Italian, expressing my sorrow at having to cancel our accommodation bookings. I mentioned that I was a student of the Italian language and was crushed at the thought of not being able to visit 'la bella Italia' and—among other delights—practise my lingual skills.

In response, I received a letter from Paolo, who would have been our B&B host in Milano, stating that he was a teacher who taught, among other subjects, the Italian language and that he missed teaching so much that in the lockdown he would like to teach me—if I would accept him as my teacher. Oh, wow! My teacher Alessandro had got away safely to his hometown of Asti, and I was over the moon at the thought of being able to continue my lessons with someone who knew how to teach.

Paolo and I write to each other every week, sharing news and views. He has a literary and historical bent of mind, as I do, so we are able to discuss a variety of subjects—like the origins of the Gregorian chant, the philosophy of Socrates and Buddha, our mutual atheism, the importance of Shakespeare in the tradition of drama, the benefits of observing fasts such as during Ramzan...

I write to him in Italian; he answers my letters also in Italian, adding news about himself, his wife and his love for sailing (he is writing a manual about safety at sea and chafing at the lockdown that keeps him away from his boat in Genoa), and then copies the text of my letter, marked with corrections in typical professorial style. I'm happy, he's happy—and my Italian has improved by the proverbial leaps and bounds.

I know no greater happiness than when he marks one of my turns of phrase with the words, '*Molto bene. Complimenti*!'

Pandemic 2120: A Love Story

Anuradha Kumar

She saw the lights zooming in on her from far away and felt fear surge through her. He was here earlier than expected. Maybe his shuttle now took less time, the engines able to take full advantage of the interplanetary winds. After all, he had been working on improving the speed resistance ratio for the last several months. He would surprise her, he had said. But this was the last thing she wanted.

She heard the pinging on her screen, and there was his face, just as she remembered. But it took just a few seconds more to make out the new scars on his face; his green hair now had shades of red and grey in it. 'That's the second surprise,' he said, his metal fingers reaching up to his hair. 'You should not be here,' she said, her tone flat and expressionless.

Any moment now, she expected the intruder alarm to go off. If his shuttle were seen, once it had breached the city's cloud shield, the drones would be out. They would attack first, the sting rays piercing his shuttle, eviscerating it in seconds, before he even had a chance to defend himself. 'There's a pandemic on,' she was trembling, suddenly unable to breathe, 'don't you ever read?' She reached for her oxygen, took it in deep gulps. And he spoke, in that metallic staccato voice she so loved, 'I have heard about that.'

'They think it's being brought in by visitors like you. Didn't you hear of the camps in the desert? And now in a city like Excalibur, they are not even allowing that. Shoot the alien first. You must not land.'

She spoke in a rush, but there was no way he could, of course. The landing decks on the buildings would open up, swallowing him and his landing shuttle, crunching everything to pieces. He would be reduced to scraps and ashes, leaving behind only his trans-modified heart and specialised brain.

'Go away,' she reached closer and whispered into the mouthpiece, endearments and the special code, in the language she had picked up.

'I have no fuel left.'

But he could not finish. She saw his face become a blur.

The alarm sirens soon blew over the island, the island that was her home. It had been a city once, one of the centres when the last epidemic had broken out a century ago. And now it was a city floating out into the sea, like the world's other big cities. Faced with rising water levels, they were now swirling, perpetually moving islands, aided by the towers of underwater motors that used helium oil from Jupiter to keep them afloat. The cities were adrift and yet well protected.

His face became fuzzy, disappeared into pixels. Panic-stricken now, she fiddled with the buttons, banged the screen, feeling like one of those tech dinosaurs she had seen in the old movies. But she could not find him. He did not reappear.

An hour later, she received the summons to a security meeting called by the town council responsible for keeping the city safe. That was how her affair with Rebus XVI, half man-half Uranian came to light.

The orders had to be followed, there were no exceptions. She would be taken to a camp, for having illicit relations at a critical time with a no-man Uranian. It would be a journey inland to a country that had once been the United States. On the way in her cable car swinging on the low-lying cables, over the Earth she saw buses. Domed bug-like vehicles that had not changed for decades. They were carrying the people she had read about, but rarely seen. The ordinary workers who like in the pandemic she had read about a century ago, were the ones who had actually built the cities, the buildings taller than ever before, and the swinging, zigzagging roads. The buildings with their solar windows, landing decks, the jetties that could stretch out to sea, the retractable roofs, the gardens, and swimming pools still needed workers and they were always being built. Even now, the workers were moving from one camp to another, like they had been for years and decades before. The buses moved slowly along the expressways that were the old, steel bands that still cut across the country. She remembered the photos handed down from one digital pod to another. The roads, the motels, and the grasslands that had stretched into the interior, where there was desert now.

The workers built the cities and towns and suburbs as everywhere; the Earth was swamped with an unending heat and in the interior of continents, the perpetual dust storms. She passed cities in their immense spherical domes built to regulate temperatures. Along one stretch were glass-shaped boxes that contained the farms, where the vital life-preserving grain and other modified vegetables were grown. She saw the moving towers, their steel blades flashing in the sun, as her cable car passed. She saw the cable cars ahead, tinted glasses meant she could never look at those inside. Sometimes they stopped at wayside stations. There were very few people. The pandemic had forced everyone in. Even the malls that must stretch beyond the high-gated towering buildings, were closed. When she finally stopped, a voice came over the speaker, one only she could hear. Station fifteen twenty-six. Around three hours away. Please disembark with care.

She had her phone, nothing else. Not her computer walkie-talkie, nor her essential vision-regulating goggles. She did not dare get in contact with Rebus. She was sure they were monitoring her gestures, her every expression. Everything would be held against her. She would never give him away.

A hundred years ago, she remembered the story she had been told. The time her great-grandfather had been in the hospital and they spoke to him only via the old-fashioned iPad. It was for love, to keep him safe. A love that had made them shun any physical intimacy. It had lasted for so long that it had become a habit. The pandemic had not just led to meaningless deaths, including that of her great-grandfather when he was only forty, but had led to strictures about everything. Movement and precaution and even about how people became physically intimate. The elaborate sanitising requirements that her grandmother would tell her about. How difficult it had been, and how quickly it became a routine.

Now for love, she had to keep Rebus away. Her only hope was that once the pandemic had eased, the restrictions had lifted, they would get the permission to marry. But the suspicions now ran too deep, especially against aliens like him. At the last united planetary meeting of scientists, they had been told of the rumours that had only gathered strength. That the illness had not come from a faulty gene in the grain strain, but a seed brought in from one of the space cities beyond the Kuiper Belt. The gene had mutated into something else, far more deadly. And everyone was accusing someone else, and the Uranians were easy to blame.

In her days at quarantine, when she lost count of time, and the time the lights faded everywhere, sometimes she would look up. One night, or it could have been early evening, she saw a light whizzing past, like a fast-moving, elusive comet. It was, she thought, perhaps the government, keeping an eye.

But she could never be sure. One day she read the news about aliens being barred for an indefinite length of time. Those still detained on Earth would board spaceships to take them away.

Many nights later, when she knew she was slowly losing her memory, she saw the purple light in the sky. Letters formed on every cloud, someone writing a message. She almost laughed. With an ache, a memory jolt, she remembered an old story. An ancestor from India who had written about leaving a message outside a lover's window, leaving the road strewn with flowers. It seemed impossible that such a demonstration was possible in these days of surveillance. But there it was, written in neon, across the thick nimbus clouds overhead. 'My darling, I have come for you.'

She knew it could be a trap. She knew she had spent so long in the desert and these were possible delusions. Of late, she had returned to the past so often, things she barely knew. She longed so often for the things everyone said had been forgotten. Simple food, the simple and ordinary gestures of love.

Wheat Fields

Tsering Gellek

blue bird fly
and soothe the sky
of her long afternoon.
think of the wind
and how
your wings will brush her cheeks
and paint them pink
and quiet the grasses.
beautiful wheat fields
you've finished growing, so they say.
so now you must be cut and harvested
taken by hand,
lifted once again into the wind
your seeds scattered here and there.

Love in the Time of Corona

Amit Dasgupta

I cannot remember the day of the week, date or time when it invaded our minds and became the central focus of our thoughts and conversations. Was it in the early hours of the morning, sometime in the month of March, or could it have been late in the evening or perhaps, it was at the dead of night? I can't truly remember though I ought to because God knows that after the first cases in Wuhan and its rapid spread, almost with fanfare and beating of drums, the virus had announced it was going to become a pandemic, sparing none. It had no intention of coming surreptitiously like a thief in the night or as the quiet plague. It came just like hunger does, and poverty, with fair warning. Yet, it was unlike the marauding locusts because this one you could not see coming but only what it left behind.

That large numbers of people died and continue to die is a constantly galloping statistic. Infection, contagion, lockdown, social distancing, quarantine became today's vocabulary. And death. WhatsApp worked overtime with reports, analysis, toll, critiques, songs of hope and bad jokes.

An erudite article in a scientific journal was rubbished by another. Jubilation at the discovery of an antidote was soon cast aside by reports of its ineffectiveness. In the slums and shanty towns, the contagion spread rapidly. With the economy shut down and livelihoods lost, the poor, as always, became the first casualties. Images of millions of stranded migrants, many barefoot, walking through the blazing sun, without food or shelter, filled our hearts with helplessness and shame. For the many who died, even the cremation was a lonely last journey. The present was grim and bleak and the future without hope. Panic and confusion became the norm. The world faced a sense of deep unease.

Nature abhors a vacuum and over centuries, humankind has been known to show extraordinary resilience especially during the darkest times. Across the globe, people were determined to rise once more. They sought out stories of solace and comfort. They learnt to rediscover suppressed and often ignored feelings, such as, respect for the simple things of life. Like humanity, for instance. And hope. And kindness. The longing for company and of laughter. The joy of reading and of music. Things they knew existed but had forgotten about.

They tried their hands at new things. In France, a person ran an entire marathon on his small balcony because he couldn't bear the thought of being cooped up in his small apartment. Some have taken to writing and reading. Many learned to cook. Some have picked up a paintbrush and easel. Almost everyone connected with their family and friends and reached out to strangers. We laughed and joked with them but more importantly, we enquired about their welfare. Several have reached out to the elderly and the infirm and the forgotten marginalised and have started to help out with community meals. This is not charity but humanity. It is who we really and truly are.

A friend, who is an amateur photographer, started to spend long hours on his terrace with a coffee, a camera and a zoom lens. He lives in the heart of Delhi with tall bushy trees that had, till now, been populated by crows, the occasional hawks and a multitude of pigeons. Over the past few days, he has photographed the grey hornbill, barbets, sunbirds, robins, parakeets, spotted owls, what looked like an eagle, and, believe it or not, the long-disappeared sparrows. They have started to return.

In a town in Kerala, the endangered Malabar civet made an appearance and was spotted on a now-empty street. Peacocks were seen dancing on the roads in Delhi. A herd of elephants went for an evening stroll in Coorg. From Jalandhar, you could see the wondrous Himalayas. Off the coast of Mumbai, whales and dolphins were sighted. In Kaziranga, a young one-horned rhino decided to check out the marketplace in the city. And loveliest of all, when you opened your window and inhaled deeply, even in Delhi, it was no longer acrid air. The rivers were clean and the sky was blue and you could hear birdsong. For the first time in months, you could see the night sky full of stars. Mother Nature was making a comeback.

But the days turned to weeks and then, into a month and more, with no real sign of respite. People started to get bored and restless and fidgety and grumpy. They craved social contact and company. Simply to *see* people is all they wanted and in fact, needed. Crowded streets, traffic jams, honking cars, queues lining up to get into shopping malls, packed elevators, loud conversations is what they missed. Being part of the hustle and bustle of modern day existence is what defined them. This new normal somehow alienated and emasculated them. They felt incomplete and alone. The lockdown started to get under their skin and doctors warned there could be an outbreak of mental health issues.

Today, we are told the virus is here to stay and that we need to learn how we should navigate around it. Life simply has to go back to normal if we are to survive, we are advised. The economic situation is disastrous. Downsizing and loss of jobs is inevitable. It is not that several entrepreneurial ventures and business would shut down but countries could, in fact, collapse under the weight of unpaid bills. We are filled with fear and a sense of foreboding. The future appears fuzzy and uncertain.

It is not long now when the civet would scurry back to its hideout and the elephants would return to the forest and we are caught up, once again, in the frenzy of today and its material expectations.

But I believe we have all been touched by something strange and perhaps, even magical. A reminder of who we really and truly are and, in fact, meant to be. Only time will tell if we would emerge kinder and gentler, that we would pause to watch the sunset, that we would reconsider our words if we feel it would cause hurt, that we would reach out to those in need and that we would respect because in doing so, we would reveal our true nature. If we do so, the Phoenix would have risen, because it must and it will.

Contributors

Jug Suraiya is a columnist, writer and the author of several fiction and non-fiction books. He can be reached at jugsuraiya@gmail.com.

Sunita Biswas is a high school teacher who is always learning. She can be reached at sunceebee@gmail.com.

Dr Nikita Bathla is a budding public health professional and advocate for health with an interest in health systems research. She can be contacted at nikita.bathla@hotmail.com.

Anjum Katyal is a writer, editor, translator and critic, who has been working in the literary, arts and culture field for close to half a century. A published poet, she also sings the blues and reviews and writes on theatre and the visual arts. She is currently Curator, NEW Festival, Santiniketan, and has been Director, Apeejay Kolkata Literary Festival.

Lakshmi Subramanian is currently professor of History at HSS, BITS Pilani, Goa campus. She has had a long and distinguished teaching and research career, and is the author of *Singing Gandhi's India Music and Sonic Nationalism*. (Roli Books, New Delhi, 2020). The article was first published in *Hindustan Times*.

Sunil Gupta is his own smorgasbord: actor, sports and TV commentator, author, bridge and tennis player. He can be contacted at sunilgupta3007@gmail.com.

Randhir Khare is a writer, poet, artist and mentor. He can be contacted at randhir.khare@gmail.com.

Deepak Sanan is a former civil servant, who believes in the constitution, unlike most institutions that are meant to uphold it! He may be contacted at deepak_sanan@hotmail.com.

Beetashok Chatterjee is an old sea dog, and the author of *Driftwood—Stories Washed Ashore*, published by Readomania. He can be contacted at chatty05@gmail.com.

Jayshree Misra Tripathi is a writer, a former Consultant, teacher and examiner in English, for the International Baccalaureate Organisation.

Dilip Bobb is a senior journalist and a writer. He has worked with the best in the business, *India Today, Indian Express, Outlook* magazine.

Sumit Mullick is a retired bureaucrat and an author.

Amrita Narayanan is a writer and psychoanalyst based in Goa. A variation of her article was first published in *Hindustan Times*.

Lalita Panicker is consulting editor, comments, *Hindustan Times*, New Delhi. She can be reached at lalita.panicker@gmail.com.

Anita Anand, with a career in development communications, is a writer, painter and therapist. Her current passions are gardening, baking and the pursuit of a more spiritual life. She can be reached at aa.comfirst@gmail.com.

Tuktuk Ghosh is a retired Indian Administrative Service Officer based in New Delhi and may be reached at tghoshk@gmail.com.

A traveller and music aficionado, **Supriya Newar**'s last book *Kalkatta Chronicles* won many hearts and much acclaim. She can be reached at connect@supriyanewar.com.

Sushmita Bose is an editor and journalist who has worked in leading publications such as *Hindustan Times*, *Business Standard* and *Khaleej Times* in New Delhi and Dubai. She's also the author of the bestselling, *Single in the City*.

Sohan Hatangadi is a grouchy retired corporate executive, now busy poking his nose in everyone else's business.

Pooja Poddar Marwah is a woman who lives for Today, each and every day.

Avijit Dutt is an actor, theatre maker and communicator. He teaches, works and lives in Delhi. He can be contacted at avijit@gmail.com.

Reena I. Puri has been weaving stories for as long as she can remember. She has penned various stories for children.

Snigdha Agrawal (nee Banerjee) enjoys writing prose, poetry, travelogues and is a regular reviewer on Tripadvisor, writing under pen name 'puchka'.

Journalist, editor and citizen of India, **Antara Dev Sen** is now not quite herself. She can be contacted at antaradevsen@googlemail.com.

Mitra Phukan is a novelist, short story writer, translator and columnist who lives in Assam.

Debi Mukhopadhyay calls herself learner unlimited. Having been a teacher, teacher trainer, English language examiner, baker (at home), traveller to remote places, she has learned about people, customs and most of all, about herself.

Jael Silliman is an author, scholar and women's rights activist.

Now retired and having discovered amateur singing for YouTube mostly in the Sindhi language, **Deepak Hiranandani** has worked at architecture, landscape, heritage conservation and the teaching of these subjects as well as freelance writing and photography.

Born and brought up in Kolkata, **Papia Roy** is a writer, editor and graphic designer, who lives with her family in the US.

Nandini Dutta is a retired professor, now teaching in an international school. She can be contacted at nandinidutta@gmail.com.

Navtej Sarna is the author of several works of fiction and non-fiction and a former Ambassador of India to the US. He can be reached at: navtej.sarna@gmail.com. His articles were published in *The Week* magazine.

J. Alfred Prufrock is an occasional traveller, chef, writer, quizzer, agony uncle, full-time father, husband and son. Also a civil servant.

Mousumi Sengupta has been a print, radio and television personality, a news anchor cum journalist. Currently, she is a part-time columnist, a social activist and a full-time helicopter mom!

Debanjan Chakrabarti's day job is that of Director of British Council in East and Northeast India. At night, he often dreams of playing at the Championships in Wimbledon or batting at Eden Gardens for India.

Mangala Gouri Chakraborty doesn't do things until she must: She writes because her dam has burst.

Amit Dasgupta is an aspiring writer. His last book *The House and Other Stories* was published by Yoda Press. He can be reached at amit.dasgupta2013@yahoo.com.

Bunny Suraiya is a novelist, editorial consultant and a writer. She can be reached at bunnysuraiya@gmail.com.

Anuradha Kumar is a writer; her most recent novel is *Coming Back to the City: Mumbai Stories* from Speaking Tiger books. *The Hottest Summer in Years* is forthcoming from Yoda Press. She can be contacted at anukumar0811@gmail.com.

Tsering Gellek was born in California and is the director of the Sarnath International Nyingma Institute.